协和医学院系列规划教材

供群医学、临床医学、公共卫生、卫生管理等专业用

（中英双语版）

群医学

Population Medicine

[新西兰] 乔纳森·格雷
Jonathon Gray

[新西兰] 卡瑞娜·麦克哈迪　著
Karina McHardy

[英] 缪尔·格雷
Muir Gray

王辰　杨维中　主译

张孔来　主审

中国协和医科大学出版社

北　京

Print ISBN 978 - 0 - 473 - 33367 - 6

Epub ISBN 978 - 0 - 473 - 33299 - 0

© by Ko Awatea 2014.

著作权合同登记：图字 01 -2020 -4827 号

图书在版编目（CIP）数据

群医学／（新西兰）乔纳森·格雷（Jonathon Gray），（新西兰）卡瑞娜·麦克哈迪（Karina McHardy），（英）缪尔·格雷（Muir Gray）著；王辰，杨维中译. —北京：中国协和医科大学出版社，2021.4

ISBN 978 - 7 - 5679 - 1550 - 3

Ⅰ.①群… Ⅱ.①乔… ②卡… ③缪… ④王… ⑤杨… Ⅲ.①卫生管理 Ⅳ.①R19

中国版本图书馆 CIP 数据核字（2021）第 021008 号

群医学

主　　译：	王　辰　杨维中
责任编辑：	雷　南　戴申倩
封面设计：	许晓晨
责任校对：	张　麓
责任印制：	卢运霞

出版发行：**中国协和医科大学出版社**

（北京市东城区东单三条 9 号　邮编 100730　电话 010 -65260431）

网　　址：	www.pumcp.com
经　　销：	新华书店总店北京发行所
印　　刷：	小森印刷（北京）有限公司

开　　本：	787mm×1092mm　1/16
印　　张：	17.25
字　　数：	235 千字
版　　次：	2021 年 4 月第 1 版
印　　次：	2023 年 7 月第 3 次印刷
定　　价：	86.00 元

ISBN 978 -7 -5679 -1550 -3

翻译团队

主译

王　辰　中国医学科学院 北京协和医学院群医学及公共卫生学院

杨维中　中国医学科学院 北京协和医学院群医学及公共卫生学院

主审

张孔来　中国医学科学院 北京协和医学院基础学院

中文版审校专家（按姓氏拼音为序）

毕振强　山东省疾病预防控制中心

崔富强　北京大学公共卫生学院

廖苏苏　中国医学科学院 北京协和医学院基础学院

乔友林　中国医学科学院 北京协和医学院群医学及公共卫生学院

单广良　中国医学科学院 北京协和医学院基础学院

唐金陵　中国科学院深圳理工大学

肖　丹　中日友好医院

杨　汀　中日友好医院

詹思延　北京大学公共卫生学院

赵方辉　中国医学科学院肿瘤医院

译者（按姓氏拼音为序）

陈秋兰　中国疾病预防控制中心

冯录召　中国医学科学院 北京协和医学院群医学及公共卫生学院

贾萌萌　中国医学科学院 北京协和医学院群医学及公共卫生学院

赖圣杰　英国南安普顿大学

冷志伟　中国医学科学院 北京协和医学院群医学及公共卫生学院

李晋磊　中国医学科学院 北京协和医学院群医学及公共卫生学院

宁桂军　中国疾病预防控制中心

苏琪茹　深圳儿童医院

苏小游　中国医学科学院 北京协和医学院群医学及公共卫生学院

佟训靓　北京医院

王　辰　中国医学科学院 北京协和医学院群医学及公共卫生学院

杨维中　中国医学科学院 北京协和医学院群医学及公共卫生学院

伊赫亚　中华预防医学会

张　娟　中国医学科学院 北京协和医学院群医学及公共卫生学院

张　婷　中国医学科学院 北京协和医学院群医学及公共卫生学院

张惺惺　中国医学科学院 北京协和医学院群医学及公共卫生学院

张　敏　中国医学科学院 北京协和医学院群医学及公共卫生学院

赵　健　中国医学科学院 北京协和医学院群医学及公共卫生学院

译者的话
Translators' Preface

国际学界将群医学（population medicine）定义为由卫生保健系统自身或者联合其他协作者，在实现个体保健及治疗的基础上，为促进人口整体健康水平而开展的一系列具体活动。2014 年，牛津大学缪尔·格雷（Muir Gray）爵士、新西兰学者乔纳森·格雷（Jonathon Gray）和卡瑞娜·麦克哈迪 (Karina McHardy) 共同编著了 *Population Medicine* 一书。为向读者介绍国外群医学的理念、方法和技能，我们引进并组织翻译了该著作。

《群医学》一书分为三部分。第一部分"平衡各项责任——厘清群医学的目标"，介绍临床医生新的责任、人群健康、患者体验和价值提升等与群医学相关的概念和理念，是后两部分的理论基础；第二部分"群医学的基本要素"，讲述在服务体系、组织和文化角度如何构建群医学的基本要素，是从管理视角指导群医学实践的部分；第三部分"发展群医学技能"，阐述在领导力、照护质量、知识管理和预算制订方面如何提升工作技能，是从个人视角指导群医学实践的部分。

由于该书作者所处的社会环境和卫生体系，以及该书所用的特定词汇和语义语境与我国不尽相同，内容又涉及众多相关学科，翻译或难达意，甚或存在错误。为帮助学习，我们适当增加了译者注释，并采用原文与译文双语对应排版的方式，便于读者对照原文准确领悟作者原意，也欢迎读者发现并向译者指出翻译中的问题。

2019 年初，王辰、单广良教授等将群医学学科列为协和医学院的重点建设发展学科，并向北京市教育委员会申请高校高精尖学科建设项目，于同年 5 月获得批准。6 月，国务院学位委员会批准协和医学院增设交叉学科"群医学"。2020 年 7 月 14 日，王辰、杨维中、单广良和冷志伟在《中华医学杂志》发表了述评《群医学：弥合预防医学与临床医学裂痕的新兴学科》。同年 7 月 16 日，协和医学院正式成立群医学及公共卫生学院，拉开了中国群医学学科建设的序幕。

群医学的理论在实践中不断地发展。引进国外的理论和理念，不仅为了借鉴，更要体现学术精髓，有所创新发展。2019 年以来，我国在群医学领域开展了大量理论研究和实践，不断地发展和完善群医学的概念与内涵。

群医学理念引进我国之初，在学界曾引起广泛的讨论，其中讨论的主要问题之一是"population medicine"一词的翻译。一些专家提出翻译为"人群医学"或"群体医学"。我们之所以译为群医学，是为了更能体现"population"的全部内涵，即被医学照护和施予医学照护双方之群：不仅仅包括已经就诊的和还没有就诊但需要医学救治、照护的人群（患者之群），处于发生某种疾病高风险状态的人群（高风险者之群），需要预防疾病发生、基本健康的人群（常人之群），还包含医学卫生工作者（医者之群）以及与群医学相关的众多学科（学科之群）、实施群医学指导下的公共卫生行动的社会各界（界别之群）。群医学这门学科帮助医务人员改变以往主要关注个体健康的行为观念，开始注重以"群"之方法关注"群"之健康，从医学角度统筹调动各方资源和能力，指导公共卫生实践。协和医学院群医学及公共卫生学院希望在这样的价值观和理念指引下，集各学科之优势，聚社会各群体之参与，发展群医学学科，践行群医学理念，促进形成"健康入万学万策万行，万学万策万行务健康"的局面，推动我国实现从"以个体治病为中心"向"以人民健康为中心"的伟大转变。

根据目前的研究进展，**协和医学院将群医学定义为：群医学是融合、运**

用当代医学及相关学科的知识和原理，基于现实可及的卫生资源条件，统筹个体卫生行为与群体卫生行动，指导公共卫生实践，实现人群整体与长远健康效益最大化的一门新兴的医学交叉学科。

《群医学》双语本可作为群医学、临床医学、公共卫生、卫生管理等专业本科生、研究生或研修生的教材或教学辅助资料，或供相关领域的教学人员、研究人员参考使用。

希望群医学的研究、教学和实践能够促进社会文明进步，增益广大人民健康福祉。

王　辰　杨维中
于北京东单北极阁三条 31 号
2021 年 4 月

Foreword

We are committed to writing a series of books together, as primers in the toolkit of health transformation.

The healthcare system does not sit in 'splendid isolation': it exists within wondrous complexity. The emergent science of complexity is now required knowledge for all health workers interested in making the right change, in the right way. The health system is 'complex' with a great many independent parts interacting with each other in a great many ways. Thus we see spontaneous self-organisation – adaptive systems that latch on to advantage – and the emergence of new states from the creativity that resides at the interface between systems and the surrounding chaos.

In this series, we are working with a variety of experts to unpack the toolkit needed to make transformative change within this complex environment. This is a task we know we share because, for all health workers, there is a simple equation that makes transformation essential: increasing demand and increasing costs in a context of limited budgets.

At Counties Manukau Health, a District Health Board serving a diverse population of more than 500,000 in South Auckland, New Zealand, we call this challenge 'Achieving a Balance'.

Isolated service or process improvements are not enough and can only delay the day when we will run out of beds. Scaling-up of individual projects has little impact on such a complex challenge.

Of course, we do need to keep improving our current services, but we must also equip ourselves to address the complex challenges ahead. This means learning how to design and implement both system integrations and whole-of- system change that transform the way we deliver, and people experience, care.

我们致力于共同撰写一套丛书，作为医疗保健转型工具包的入门读物。

医疗保健系统不会与世隔绝、岿然独立，而是与复杂奥妙的外部环境共存；对于所有希望以正确方式做出正确改变的医疗工作者来说，新兴的复杂性科学是必备知识。医疗卫生系统是"复杂的"，其中许多独立部分以多种方式相互影响。因此，我们看到了自发的自组织——发挥优势的自适应系统——以及来自系统与混沌界面的创造力所产生的新状态。

在本丛书中，我们与多位专家合作，开发了这套在复杂环境中进行变革转型所需的工具包。这是我们共同的任务，因为对于所有医疗卫生工作者而言，一个简单的算式解释了转型的不可或缺：在预算有限的情况下，需求和成本正日趋增加。

在新西兰南奥克兰的马努考郡卫生局——一个为超过 50 万人口提供医疗照护的地区健康委员会——我们将这种挑战称为"实现平衡"。

单纯地改善医疗服务或流程还远远不够，也只能推迟医院床位不足那一天的到来。扩大单个项目规模对于应对如此复杂的挑战也仅如蚍蜉撼树。

当然，我们确实需要不断提升现有医疗服务，但我们也必须使自己具备应对未来复杂挑战的能力。这意味着要学习如何设计和实施系统整合和全系统变革，这将改变医疗的提供方式以及人们的体验和照护方式。

This is why we have established our innovation and improvement institute, Ko Awatea, with its dual tasks of 'improving and transforming today'. For both tasks, a deep understanding of complexity, large-scale change, systems and systems thinking are crucial.

We are collaborating together, and working closely with local colleagues on this series of digital books to develop our collective transformation capabilities.

We believe that population medicine is a new responsibility for the 21st century. At Counties Manukau Health, we look at our responsibilities through a lens of the 'Triple Aim'[1] of keeping people well, improving patient experience, and affordability. Hospital care is an expensive and over-used setting for delivering services and it is a responsibility we share with our entire population to reduce demand through whole-of-system change.

In this book, we identify the changing responsibility of the manager and the clinician in an era in which healthcare is funded by the whole population and not just by the patients who see doctors. Together, we explore the dual responsibility of clinicians and managers to patients and whole populations, and the actions they need to take to discharge that responsibility.

To effect the transformational change our population needs and deserves, we firmly believe we must embrace the complementary sciences of improvement, large-scale change, and complexity so that we can design innovatively and act our way to an excellent and sustainable future. This book on population medicine is an important piece of the knowledge and skills 'toolkit' we will need to bring about the change we want and need.

Jonathon Gray and Muir Gray

---

[1] The IHI Triple Aim. Institute for Healthcare Improvement Website. www.ihi.org/offerings/Initiatives/TripleAim.Accessed 15 July 2014.

这就是我们为什么建立了寇·阿瓦提（Ko Awatea）创新与改进研究所，其承担着"进行当下的改进与转型"的双重任务。针对这两项任务，深刻理解复杂性、大规模变革、体系和系统思维都至关重要。

我们和研究所一起，与本地同事密切合作，开发出这一系列数字书籍，以发展我们的协同转型能力。

我们相信，群医学是21世纪的医学新职责。在马努考郡卫生局，我们从"三重目标"①的角度看待这份职责，即保持人群健康、改善患者体验，让医疗价格合理。医院是可以提供照护的机构，但价格昂贵且已被过度使用。通过制度改革来减少需求，是我们与全体人民的共同责任。

在本书中，我们发现，在医疗保健由全人群而不仅是就诊患者提供资金支持的时代中，管理者和临床医生的责任正在不断发生变化。我们共同探讨了临床医生和管理者对患者和全人群的双重职责，以及他们为履行这一责任的需要采取的行动。

为了实施我们的人群所需和应有的转型变革，我们坚信：我们必须吸纳改善所需的其他科学，相信大规模变革是大势所趋，意识到医疗保健系统所处环境的复杂性，以便我们能够设计创新，并为实现美好和可持续的未来而努力。这本有关群医学的书是实现我们必要变革所需知识和技能"工具包"的重要部分。

乔纳森·格雷

缪尔·格雷

---

① 2007年，医疗卫生保健改善研究所（IHI）开发了一个框架，用于卫生保健系统使用各种指标优化绩效。由于该框架采用"三管齐下的方法"，IHI称之为三重目标（triple aim），即人群健康（population health），卫生保健服务体验（experience of care）和人均成本（per capita cost）。

Preface

This series is about healthcare transformation and the large-scale change we need to implement within a highly complex system. Central to that transformation is our vision of keeping people well, improving patient experience, and affordability. We have been helped by the inspirational concept of the 'Triple Aim', promoted by our colleagues at the Institute for Healthcare Improvement.

We started with Creating Systems (Book 1) to highlight both the nature of the problem and the source of the solution. In that book, the focus is on the shift from 'two-box' (primary-secondary) healthcare to 'four-box' integrated systems of care, or 'care pathways'. We have expanded the focus to acknowledge that, optimally, healthcare systems need to be components of cross sector-integrated health systems the purpose of which is to promote health and reduce the incidence of ill-health. Later in the series, we will delve into two crucial contributors to the success of any complex organisational system in Creating Culture (Book 3) and Knowledge Management (Book 4), before exploring what we can learn from examples of Triple Value Healthcare (Book 5). In this book, Population Medicine (Book 2), we highlight and clarify the importance of population medicine to the healthcare transformation before us all. We also highlight how you, as a health professional, can discharge your current responsibilities confidently while identifying opportunities to transform the system you are serving.

Our District Health Board has a responsibility for the health and wellness of our entire population. That is not a universal situation, and healthcare now has the opportunity to explore the responsibilities of working at a population level, as well as at the level of the hospital or the individual patient. This book is intended for a

前 言
Preface

本系列丛书内容涉及医疗保健转型以及在高度复杂系统中实施的大规模变革。变革的核心就是我们的愿景，即保持人群健康、改善患者体验以及让医疗价格合理。医疗卫生保健改善研究所的同事提倡的"三重目标"这一概念激发了我们的灵感。

《创建体系》（第一册）是整套丛书的起点，着重强调问题的本质和解决方案的来源。在此书中，关注重点从"两盒式"（初级－二级）医疗保健转向"四盒式"整合医疗保健系统或"医疗保健路径"。我们还对重点进行了拓展，承认医疗保健系统最好是跨部门整合型医疗系统的组成部分；这种整合型系统的目的是促进健康并减少健康问题的发生率。在丛书的后半部，我们将深入探讨任何复杂性组织系统取得成功的两个关键因素，即《创建文化》（第三册）和《知识管理》（第四册），随之是《医疗保健的三重目标》（第五册）中的案例学习。在《群医学》（第二册）这本书中，我们强调并阐明了群医学在当前医疗保健转型中的重要性。我们还强调，一名医疗卫生保健专业人士如何能够自信地履行当下职责，同时寻找机会以改进所工作的系统。

我们的地区卫生健康委员会对整个地区人群的健康和福祉负责。这不是一个普遍状况，但医疗保健现在有机会探索在人群、医院或患者个体各个层面所承担的相应责任。本书的广大读者群包括临床医生、资助者、管理者、

broad audience of clinicians, funders, managers, public health practitioners, politicians, and others. Some specific content will be more relevant to certain professional groups than others, but we believe the core messages of the book are relevant to all.

As Muir Gray once said:

> *Population medicine is a 21st century necessity and we need bilingual clinicians, those who can speak the language of their specialty and the language of healthcare for populations.*

We think the challenge now is to be multilingual – languages of both personalised and population medicine, in the context of specialist and more generalist skills, within an environment of complexity requiring cross-sector collaboration, networking, and understanding of change at scale.

This is not a cry of despair – public health colleagues and others have long guided us into these fields of study – but the future requires every healthcare worker to engage with the health languages of the future. We hope you enjoy learning these new languages!

Jonathon Gray and Karina McHardy

公共卫生从业人员、政界人士及其他人士在内。一些特定内容将更适用于某些专业团体，但是我们认为本书的核心内容适用于所有人。

正如缪尔·格雷曾经说过的：

> "群医学是 21 世纪的必需品，我们需要会'双语'的临床医生，他们既可以说自己专业的语言，也可以说人群医疗保健的语言。"

我们认为现在的挑战是在兼具专科和全科的技能背景下，也在需要跨部门合作、建立工作网络和理解大规模变革复杂性的环境中，要会"多语"——即个性化医学和群医学的语言。

这不是绝望的呐喊——虽然公共卫生同行和其他人长期以来一直在引导我们进入这些研究领域——但是未来要求每一位医疗保健从业人员都必须使用未来的卫生保健语言。我们希望您享受学习这些新语言！

乔纳森·格雷
卡瑞娜·麦克哈迪

Contents

目　　录

Part 1

Balancing responsibilities – clarifying the goal of population medicine

第 1 章
平衡各项责任——厘清群医学的目标

1.1 Population medicine – a new responsibility for the 21st century

In this section, we explore:
- *why clinicians feel their sole responsibility lies with the patient in front of them, a situation that arose from an era when the patient paid the doctor directly*
- *the new responsibility of the clinician to and for the whole population and the actions clinicians need to take to discharge that responsibility*

■ The traditional responsibility of doctors

Since Hippocrates, the traditional responsibility that doctors have felt is to the patient in front of them either on the other side of the desk or lying in bed.

This responsibility entailed complete loyalty to the individual patient, and a commitment of resources without consideration of cost.

In practice, clinicians have become accustomed to limiting the use of one resource to individual patients in order to ensure that it is available to all. This finite resource that the clinician limits so that all patients might benefit is time. If a clinician did not limit the time given to one patient, there would be no time for other patients – indeed, clinicians would rarely get home. This practice has persisted for years despite the knowledge that not only many of a clinician's patients want more time but also that some patients would report a better outcome if more time had been invested in their care. It could be argued that clinicians have not rationed their time with sufficient rigour and, as a consequence, have suffered burnout, a problem that will become more common as the pressure on resources for healthcare intensifies.

■ Deriving greater value from resources

Although time is finite, the benefits of face-to-face time can be enhanced, for example, by using online resources to extend the consultation. Although money is also finite, unlike time it cannot be extended in the same way. Money is inelastic: money spent on one patient cannot be spent on another. Thus, if care is to be extended to patients other than those already being seen by a busy service, greater value will need to be derived from existing resources. This represents a new challenge, entailing new responsibilities for clinicians.

> *What are the new responsibilities of the clinician who must continue to remain focused on the needs and demands of an individual patient but must also take account of patients not yet in contact with the service?*
>
> *How do these new responsibilities relate to the traditional responsibility of doctors?*

第1节　群医学——21世纪的新责任

在本节中，我们将会探讨：

- 为什么临床医生认为自己只需要对诊治的患者负责？这源于患者直接向医生付费的时代。
- 临床医生应当对整个人群承担新责任，并付诸行动。

■ 传统意义上医生的责任

从希波克拉底时代起，医生就认为他们只需要向自己诊疗的患者负责。

这种传统责任要求医生全身心救治每名患者，保证资源充足，无需考虑成本。

在实践中，临床医生们已经习惯尽可能减少在个体患者身上花费的时间，以确保所有患者都能得到诊治。时间资源有限，限制个人配额能让所有患者获益。如果临床医生不限制单个患者的诊疗时间，那么其他患者就将无法获得应有的诊疗时间，并且医生自己也无法下班回家。虽然许多患者都希望获得更多的诊疗时间，而且这样会让他们感觉诊疗效果更好，但是限制患者诊疗时间的做法已经持续多年。可以说，不能严格地分配时间不仅让医生精疲力竭，随着医疗资源紧缺的压力加剧，这个问题还将使变得更加普遍。

■ 从资源中获取更多价值

虽然医生的时间有限，但是可以通过采取其他措施增加面对面沟通的获益，例如可以通过在线形式拓展咨询的时间或范围。金钱也是有限的，但金钱是与时间不相同的资源，其收益无法使用类似措施进行扩展。金钱同样缺乏灵活性：为一名患者所花的费用不能再转移到另一名患者身上。因此，如果要使已经满负荷运转的医疗系统服务更多的人群，就需要从现有资源中获取更多价值。这是新挑战，也势必成为临床医生的新职责。

临床医生必须继续关注个体病人的需要和需求，但也必须同时关注那些还没有接受服务的病人。在这种情况下，临床医生的职责是什么？

这些新职责与医生的传统职责有什么关系？

■ The changing contractual position of doctors

In the 20th century, it was argued that the doctor's responsibilities were to the individual patient in a consultation and to that patient alone. Until 1948, doctors in the United Kingdom received their income directly from the patient sitting in front of them. This simple contractual arrangement is shown in Figure 1.1. For doctors in some other countries, this is still the contractual position today.

In the general practice setting in New Zealand, there is a part payment from the patient, with the majority of the cost met from general taxation and passed on via capitation funding to general practitioners.

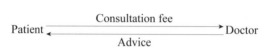

Figure 1.1   The 'direct' contractual arrangement between doctor and patient

In many countries, however, the contractual relationship between doctors and patients has changed (see Figure 1.2). For the majority of services, people are no longer prevented from accessing care by its cost because the resources for care are provided by the whole population. Of those people providing the resources for care, some:

- *are patients already in contact with the service*
- *have the condition (i.e. are in need) but have not yet made contact with the service*
- *are healthy and will never develop the condition (i.e. not in need)*

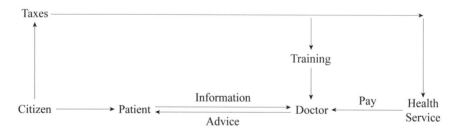

Figure 1.2   The new contractual relationship between doctors and patients

With the exception of the United States of America (USA), this contractual arrangement exists in every developed country, although it is possible that the USA is now on the way to complete coverage of its population.

In other settings including New Zealand, this change in contractual arrangement had disadvantages.

- *Some doctors no longer acted as if the 'customer was king' and treated patients with less respect*
- *Few doctors regarded themselves as the stewards of public resources and*

■ 医患合同关系的不断变化

在 20 世纪，医生的职责只针对个体患者，而且只需要对诊治的患者负责即可。1948 年以前，英国医生直接向诊治的患者收费。图 1.1 展示了这种简单的合同关系。在某些国家中，这种医患之间仍在沿用这种合同关系。

在新西兰的全科医疗环境中，患者需要支付部分诊疗费用，绝大多数诊疗费用由普通税收承担，并通过按人头付费的方式支付给全科医生。

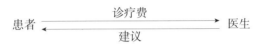

图 1.1　医生和患者之间的"直接"合同关系

但是，在许多国家和地区，医患之间的合同关系已经发生了变化（图 1.2）。大多数医疗服务系统中，所需医疗资源由全民买单，患者不再因为无法承担医疗费用而无法获得医治。为这些医疗资源买单的人群包括：

- 已经使用医疗卫生保健的患者；
- 已患病（即，有需求者）但尚未使用医疗卫生保健的患者；
- 现在健康，且永远不会患这种病的人（即，无需求者）。

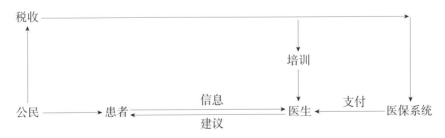

图 1.2　医生和患者之间的新型合同关系

除美国外，所有发达国家都存在这种合同契约，但是美国现在也在尝试改革，让这种合同契约逐步覆盖全部人口。

在包括新西兰在内的其他发达地区，合同契约的改变引起很多问题：

- 一些医生不再遵循"顾客是上帝"的原则，对患者变得不够尊重；
- 少数医生不再自视为公共资源的管理者，而仅承担着资源分配者的角

acted merely as the dispensers of resources. One NHS medical manager remarked it was as if doctors were writing a cheque in the supermarket but thought that their bank was going to pay, not their own account.

■ Medical management – responsibility and accountability for a service

In the last decade of the 20th century, new responsibilities for clinicians were articulated, for patient safety, quality of care, and resource management.

Many clinicians, however, were unwilling to accept the responsibility for managing resources, leaving only a small proportion of clinicians to become medical managers. Of those clinicians who accepted the role, most were part- time, but some became full-time medical directors or chief executives of a hospital (see Figure 1.3).

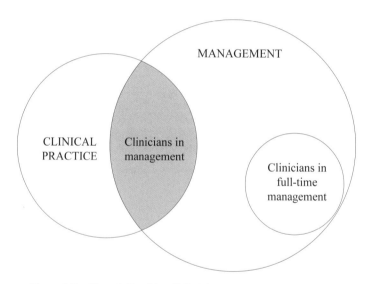

Figure 1.3   The relationship of clinicians to resource management

■ Population medicine – accountability to and for a population

In the 21st century, the responsibilities of a clinician continue to include loyalty and commitment to the well-being of an individual patient and to the quality and safety of the care they provide. These responsibilities are now complemented and supplemented by a new responsibility to the population that provides the resources for care.

The population that provides the resources for care contains the patients who are already being treated, but for every long-term condition it also includes other people with the condition who have not yet been referred. Furthermore, the population that made the decision to allocate the resources for healthcare has done so having decided that those resources will produce more value from healthcare than if they were invested in education, state pensions, defence, or any other public service.

色。一位英国国家医疗服务体系（National Health Service，NHS）医疗管理者描述，这就好比医生在超市里开支票，他们认为这钱是由银行来支付而不是花自己的账户上的钱。

■ 医疗管理——服务的职责与义务

在 20 世纪最后十年里，患者安全、医疗质量和资源管理被明确纳入临床医生的职责范畴。

然而，只有一小部分临床医生成为医疗管理者，大多数临床医生不愿承担资源管理的责任。在接受了管理者角色的临床医生中，大多数人以兼职身份同时开展临床实践与资源管理，但是也有一部分临床医生成为专职医疗主管或医院的首席执行官（图 1.3）。

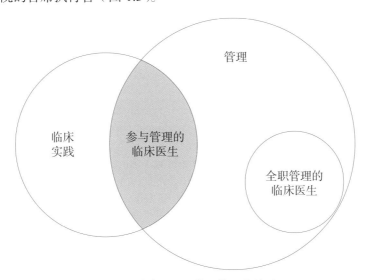

图 1.3 临床医生和资源管理的关系

■ 群医学：对人群、为人群承担的责任义务

在 21 世纪，临床医生的职责继续包括全心全意治疗每个患者、以患者福祉为己任，为他们提供安全合格的卫生保健服务。但是现在这些已经被新职责所补充替代，即需要对医疗卫生保健资源。

临床医生既需要为已在接受治疗和长期有卫生服务需求的患者提供资源，也需要为没有转诊到卫生服务体系接受服务的患者提供资源。此外，那些决定将资源分配给医疗卫生保健的民众认为，与投资教育、养老、国防或者任何其他公共服务相比，将这些资源投入医疗卫生保健服务会获取更多的收益。

With resources always being limited, by choosing to implement one option, there is a benefit forgone as resources are then not available for other options. The lost benefit from the next best use of the resources is the opportunity cost. (1)

The good management of resources by a medical manager is of obvious benefit to the population, but population medicine entails more than resource management. Clinicians in the 21st century are expected to act as stewards of the allocated resources, and to become conscious not only of the people who could benefit from healthcare or who are already in receipt of this benefit, but also of the 'benefit foregone' by the whole population such as the education of children or the amelioration of poverty.

The concept of stewardship has a long history: originally it concerned the administration of an estate on behalf of the lord of the manor. More recently, the concept carries connotations of a deeper responsibility that has arisen from the concept's use in the context of environmental sustainability, for example:

Stewardship is to hold something in trust for another. (2)

There are calls for a broader perspective to be taken in clinical practice, one that takes into account not only the patient's clinical condition – personalisation – but also the patient's values and the environment in which they live – contextualisation. In parallel, an even broader perspective is required when considering a health service with responsibility for and accountability to not only the patients in contact with the service – the traditional role of the clinician as medical manager – but also the whole population of people in need (Figure 1.4). Furthermore, there must be an accountability to the population that has provided the resources for care.

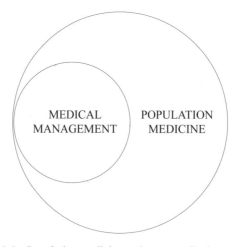

Figure 1.4   Population medicine embraces medical management

资源总是有限的，选择将资源投入一个领域，其他领域就无法利用这笔资源了，这样就会造成收益损失。这种以我们认为最有效利用资源的形式取代先前形式造成的收益损失，就是机会成本[1]。

医疗管理者如果能够很好地管理资源，会明显改善人群的健康效益；但是，群医学对资源管理者的要求却并非止步于此。21 世纪的临床医生应该成为真正意义的资源管家（stewards）——他们不仅要了解谁将会从卫生保健中获益，谁已经获益；还需要认识到资源分配给全人群医疗卫生保健带来的机会成本，如在儿童教育、消除贫困等方面带来的损益（benefit foregone）。

"管家职权"（stewardship）的概念有悠久的历史：起初这个词主要表示代表庄园主管理庄园的工作。现在，这个概念在可持续发展背景下，衍生出更深层次的责任：

"管家职权"就是受他人委托掌管某物[2]。

现在都在呼吁从更广阔的视角审视临床实践，这不仅要考虑患者个体的临床状态（个性化），也要考虑患者的价值观和他们的生活背景（情景化）。同时，采用更广阔的视角考虑医疗卫生保健时，需要临床医生承担好作为医疗管理者的传统责任，为个体患者提供良好的诊疗照护，还应当让所有有医疗需求的人能够利用好卫生资源（图 1.4）。况且，医疗资源本由全人群提供，也必须为全人群尽责。

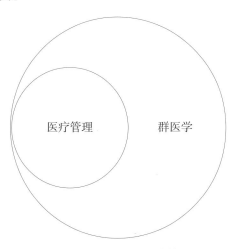

图 1.4　群医学包括医疗管理

■ Seven new responsibilities for improving population health in the 21st century

In the first decade of the 21st century, the focus of management and leadership development has been on managing an institution, whether it is a health centre or a hospital. The emphasis on quality improvement, on increasing the effectiveness of care, and on safety, also focused around institutions, has been essential, but it is not sufficient to meet the challenges of the 21st century.

Clinicians of the 21st century have a responsibility not just to the patients who happen to have made contact with their service but also for all the people whose needs could be met, directly or indirectly, by their service. In addition to achieving high levels of quality and safety, there are seven actions that need to be taken to discharge this new set of responsibilities and improve the health of populations (see Table 1.1).

Table 1.1 Discharging new responsibilities for improving population health in the 21st century

New responsibility	Action
Supporting all patients, not just those referred	Creating population-based, integrated systems
Health promotion	Preventing disease and promoting health and well-being
Equity	Ensuring fairness and justice
Outcomes	Getting the right outcomes for the right patients
Value	Getting the right patients to the right resources
Waste	Getting the right outcomes with the least waste
Sustainability	Doing the right things to protect resources for future generations

Some of these responsibilities could be seen as an extension of the clinician's responsibility to the organisation that employs them, but the first three and the last one, which are inter-related, are new. Of these new responsibilities, perhaps the most challenging is the commitment to all people in need, and not just to those people who have been referred.

From one perspective, broken legs do not pose a problem for health services. All the people with broken legs reach the right service, irrespective of the assertiveness of the patient, the patient's social status or the competence and beliefs of a general practitioner. People with cancer also tend to reach the right service, although there may be delays in the time taken to reach the service due to factors relating to the beliefs and behaviours of both patients and clinicians. For people who have one or more long-term conditions, however, many of them who

■ 21 世纪促进人群健康的七个新职责

在 21 世纪前十年，管理和领导力的研究兴趣多聚焦于管理机构，无论其为健康中心或医院。以机构为中心，提升医疗卫生保健质量、提高效益和保证患者安全是至关重要的，但这不足以应对 21 世纪的挑战。

21 世纪临床医生的职责不仅仅是为那些寻求医疗服务个体患者提供帮助，而且还应尽其所能满足所有人群直接或间接的需求。除了优质安全的服务外，还需要采取七项行动来履行这一系列的新职责，改善人群的健康状况（表 1.1）。

表 1.1　21 世纪临床医生为促进人群健康所应履行的新职责

新职责	行动
为所有患者提供支持，而不仅是就医者	构建以人群为基础的、有机整合的各类系统
健康促进	预防疾病，促进健康及福祉
公平性	确保公平与公正
结局	让每个患者都能得到合适的结局
价值	让每个患者都能获得合适的资源
浪费	以最少的浪费获取合适的效果
可持续性	做正确的事，保护资源，以利后人

这七项职责有些可看作是医生对所在工作机构的职责的延伸，但是前三个及最后一个是相互关联且全新的职责。对于这些全新的职责，也许最大的挑战是对"所有有需求的群体"而不仅仅是对那些"前来求医者"负责。

比如，腿部骨折不会对医疗卫生保健造成麻烦。因为所有腿部骨折患者都能得到妥善处治，而与患者的个人决断能力、社会地位或者全科医生自己的能力和信仰等关系不大。癌症患者也能得到妥善处治，但受到患者本身和医生的信仰行为等相关因素的影响，患者获得处治的时机可能会有所延迟。然而对于长期患有一种或多种疾病的人来说，很多人本来有可能从专科医

could benefit from the knowledge and skills of specialist services do not receive that benefit because they are not referred (see Figure 1.5). This problem is common for people with long-term conditions.

There are three possible solutions to this problem:

1. Expand the specialist service – this is rarely possible in an era of constraint

2. Clarify and implement referral criteria to reduce the size of the problem as depicted in Figure 1.5

3. Change the way of working in the specialist service such that the knowledge and skills of the specialists can be made available, either directly or indirectly, to all the patients who could benefit (i.e. all those in need). This is likely to be a much larger number than those currently being seen by the specialist service; at present, specialist service resources can be accessed only by a patient visiting healthcare real estate.

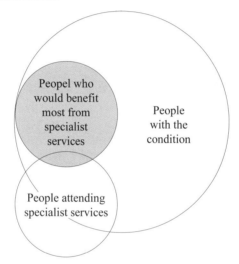

Figure 1.5   The relationship between need and supply

The changes outlined in point 3 above need to be delivered by clinicians working according to the new paradigm known as 'population medicine'.

■ What is different about population medicine?

Population medicine is a style of clinical practice or a way of working. It does not replace other paradigms, such as evidence-based medicine or patient-centred care. Instead it complements and supplements them. When clinicians practising population medicine see individual patients, they continue to use best current evidence and be patient-centred, but they also need to address the root causes of failures in the quality of care. This is best demonstrated by considering the questions clinicians might ask themselves while reflecting on the day's clinic (see Display 1.1). The clinician with a traditional approach asks a different set of questions from that posed by the clinician with a population-medicine perspective.

生的知识和技能中获益，但由于他们没能被及时转诊，而最终没有受益（图 1.5），此类问题在长期患病者中很常见。

此类问题有三种可能的解决方案：

1. 扩大专科诊疗范围，但是在一个资源稀缺的时代，这种可能性很小；

2. 明确并实施精准的转诊标准，以减少图 1.5 阴影部分的人群规模；

3. 改变专科医生的工作方式，以便专科知识和技能可以直接或间接地使所有患者（当需要时）从中受益；如是，其数量将远大于目前由专科医生服务的人数。目前，患者只有去医疗机构就诊才能接触到各种专科医疗资源。

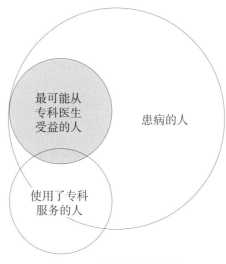

图 1.5　需求和供给的关系

想要做到第三点，临床医生就要考虑根据"群医学"实施新的范式。

■ 群医学有何不同？

群医学是一种临床实践形式或一种工作方式。群医学并非要取代其他工作范式，如循证医学或"以患者为中心"，而是对这些范式进行补充完善。当医生以群医学视角面对个体患者时，依旧要应用当前最佳的证据、以患者为中心开展诊疗活动，但是他们也需要透过个体患者，洞察医疗质量无法得到保证的根本原因。对此，最好的实践方法就是临床医生每天回顾和反思自己临床工作中遇到的问题。见场景 1.1。以群医学为视角的临床医生可以基

The latter perspective is based on the 'Five Whys' approach developed by the Toyota Motor Corporation.

Display 1.1 A traditional and a population approach to resolving the problems posed by the presentation of a child with asthma

Scenario: A child with asthma whose problems should have been able to be managed by the child, the child's family and the general practitioner (GP)	
Clinician restricted to the traditional responsibilities in healthcare	**Clinician fulfilling the responsibilities of population medicine**
1. Why did the child not know how to use her spacer? 2. Why did the GP refer the child when it would have been possible to resolve the problem using the local clinical guidelines?	1.Why was the GP not able to manage the child without referral? Because the GP did not follow the guidelines 2.Why did the GP not follow the guidelines? Because the GP did not know of their existence 3.Why did the GP not know of the existence of the guidelines? Because the GP was new to the area 4.Why are new GPs not informed about the existence of guidelines? Because we have no system for identifying and informing new GPs 5. Why do we not set up a process to identify new GPs and pharmacists to ensure they know about local guidelines, resources and referral protocols?

The population-medicine approach answers Question 5 by putting in place the necessary systems to prevent a recurrence of the problem.

Another approach using the Five Whys as a foundation would be to ask a different set of questions than the simple rhetorical question, 'Why did the child not know how to use her spacer?'. Here are twelve questions that a clinician practising population medicine could ask (see Display 1.2).

Display 1.2 A population approach to the root causes of why children with asthma (and their families) do not have the knowledge for good self- management

Scenario: A child with asthma who does not know how to use their spacer
1. How many children are there with asthma in the local population?
2. What proportion of children is referred to the specialist service?
3. How many are referred who could be managed by generalists, such as GPs and pharmacists?
4. How many children who should be referred are not?
5. Are we clear about our objectives, guidelines and referral criteria?

于丰田汽车公司开发的"五个为什么"工具提出一系列问题。这些问题与采用传统模式的临床医生提出问题有所不同。

场景1.1 在解决儿童哮喘问题时，传统医学和群医学的差异

情况：一个哮喘患儿，他的症状本应由该儿童、儿童的家庭和全科医生共同解决	
在医疗中坚守传统医学职责的医生	履行群医学职责的医生
1. 为什么这个儿童不知道如何使用储雾罐？	1. 为什么全科医生在不转诊的情况下，不能对该儿童哮喘实施有效的管理？因为该全科医生没有遵循相关指南
2. 一个本可以使用本地临床指南就解决的问题，为什么全科医生要把这个孩子转诊？	2. 为什么该全科医生没有遵循指南？因为全科医生不知道该指南的存在
	3. 为什么该全科医生不知道指南的存在？因为该全科医生是这个地区的新从业者
	4. 为什么没有人告知该全科医生指南的存在？因为我们没有识别新入职全科医生并告知其相关信息的系统
	5. 为什么我们不建立一个可以识别新入职的全科医生及药剂师的系统，以确保他们能够了解当地指南、资源和转诊的程序？

群医学通过建立必要的体系，解决上述第5个问题，防止类似情形再次发生。

再举一个使用"五个为什么"方法的例子。可提出一组不同的问题，而不仅是用一个简单反问句，如：为什么儿童不知道如何使用储雾罐？下面列举了一个临床医生从群医学的视角可能问到的12个问题（见场景1.2）。

场景1.2 群医学视角探索哮喘患儿（及其家庭）缺乏足够的自我管理知识的根本原因

情况：一个哮喘患儿不知道如何使用哮喘储雾罐
1. 当地人口中有多少儿童患有哮喘？
2. 有多大比例的儿童被转诊到专科治疗？
3. 被转诊的儿童有多少可以由通科人员，如全科医生、药剂师进行有效管理？
4. 有多少儿童应当被转诊而实际并没有转诊？
5. 我们是否清楚自己的目标、指南和转诊标准？

continued

6. Are all the generalists working with the local population including those most newly appointed aware of our guidelines and referral criteria?
7. Are all the people with asthma and their carers fully informed about how they can best manage their condition?
8. How good is the service for the local population when compared with services for similar populations in other localities?
9. What are the predisposing conditions for asthma, which are potentially avoidable?
10. How well is the child's home insulated?
11. Is there anything I can do in collaboration with this child's school and social services to improve the child's condition?
12. Can I use some of the healthcare budget to support housing or similar initiatives to reduce asthma admissions?

From a bureaucratic perspective, the components of a typical health service could be represented as a set of interconnected but separate boxes (see Figure 1.6).

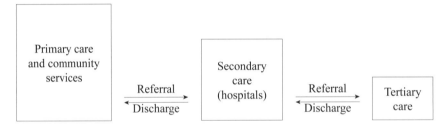

Figure 1.6   The traditional model of institutional care

There are several mis-representations regarding the depiction of reality in this figure.

- *There are large overlaps between primary and secondary care services, and between secondary and tertiary care services*
- *A hospital is portrayed as being different and distinct from 'community' services, but this perpetuates the myth that a hospital is not a community service (1)*

Another way to depict the relationship of the different types of care is as a Venn diagram (Figure 1.7), in which the different types of care are shown as a set of nested boxes, referred to as 'four-box' healthcare.

An individual may make use of all four types of care during the course of a year, or even a day, and there are 'passages' from one type of care to another. A health system designed to address inputs is shown in Figure 1.8.

For further information on effective systems, see Creating Systems (Book 1) in our Healthcare Transformation series.

续表

6. 是不是所有的全科医生（包括新入职的）都清楚指南和转诊标准？
7. 是否所有的哮喘患者及其照料者都已被告知应当如何管理他们的病情？
8. 与其他地区相比，本地区针对相似群体服务的质量如何？
9. 哮喘的促发因素是什么，哪些是可以被预防的？
10. 哮喘患儿所在住所的保温情况如何？
11. 为改善患儿的状况，我可以与儿童所在学校和社会服务机构合作做些什么？
12. 我是否能够用一些医疗卫生保健经费来支持改善住房条件或类似倡议，以减少因哮喘入院的人数？

从行政程序角度看，一个典型的医疗服务组成部分可由一组相互关联但又相互独立的单元表示（图 1.6）。

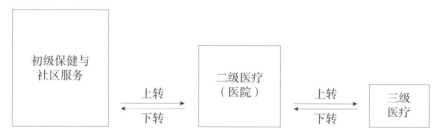

图 1.6　医疗机构患者管理的传统模式

然而，这幅图在描述现实的情况时还有不够准确之处。现实的情况是：

• 在初级和二级、二级和三级的医疗服务之间，都存在着大量重叠服务；

• 人们一般都认为，医院与"社区"医疗服务是有区别的，这加固了"医院工作不属于社区医疗服务"这一根深蒂固的观念[1]。

另一种描述不同类型医疗卫生保健之间关系的方法是用维恩图（图 1.7），图中不同类型的医疗卫生保健用一组嵌套的盒子表示，被称为"四盒式"医疗卫生保健。

一个人可以在一年甚至一天内使用四种类型的医疗卫生保健服务，而且不同类型的医疗卫生保健之间都有联结通道。图 1.8 即展示了一种旨在解决投入问题的卫生体系。

如果想更多了解有效体系的信息，请参考医疗卫生保健改革系列丛书中的《创建体系》（第一册）。

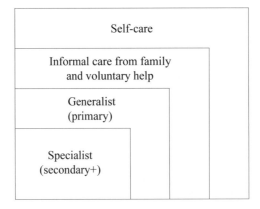

Figure 1.7　'Four-box' healthcare

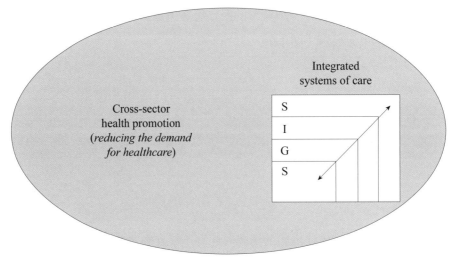

Figure 1.8　A health system designed to address inputs

Generalist and specialist partnerships

There is an increasing recognition both implicitly and explicitly that clinicians have responsibilities to the whole population as well as to the individual patient.

General practitioners have practised population medicine for decades, accepting responsibility for a defined patient population. Hospital-based specialists also have had some population responsibilities, to which they have responded to varying degrees. Some recent trends in healthcare management, for example, the separation of primary care and hospital care funding in Australia, or the development of Foundation Trusts in the English NHS, have mitigated against the exercise of responsibility for populations.

The relationship between generalists and specialists is often unnecessarily fraught for two reasons.

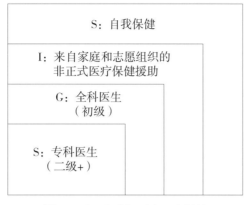

图 1.7 "四盒式"医疗卫生保健

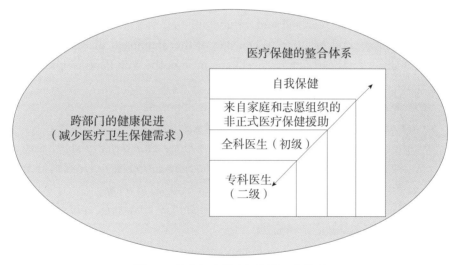

图 1.8 旨在解决投入问题的卫生体系

全科医生与专科医生的伙伴关系

人们越来越清楚地认识到，临床医生对整个人群以及患者个人都负有责任。

全科医生从事群医学已有几十年的历史，已经接受了他们需要对特定患者群体承担的责任。在医院工作的专科医生也承担了一些责任，他们对此反应不一。从近年的医疗管理趋势看，医生对人群承担的责任在不断弱化，澳大利亚初级保健资金和医院医疗资金的分离以及英国 NHS 信托基金的建立，都印证了这一趋势。

全科医生与专科医生的关系经常引起无端的困扰，其原因有以下两点：

1. Many members of both groups of clinician fail to understand the difference between the sensitivity of a symptom, sign or test result and its positive predictive value. In general practice, where the incidence and prevalence of disease is lower, the implications of the presence of a symptom, sign or positive test result is of much less concern than in specialist practice where the incidence and prevalence of the disease is much higher, principally because the generalists only refer those patients who obviously have the disease or who have a high probability of having the disease. This can mean that specialists criticise generalists for missing 'easy' diagnoses and generalists criticise specialists for over-investigation

2. There is an important difference between complex and complicated medical problems. A complex problem is epitomised by an 80-year-old woman with four diagnoses and seven prescriptions, looked after by her 50-year-old daughter who has an alcoholic husband and an unemployed son. This type of situation is standard in general practice. When one of the diagnosed diseases becomes complicated, such as heart failure developing in someone with Parkinson's disease, the generalist seeks specialist help

To maximise value for the population, it is important:

• *to help generalists and specialists work together*
• *to recognise the need to use the knowledge and skills of specialists to serve the patients in the population who have not been referred to them in addition to those patients who have been referred to them*
• *to encourage and fund specialists to apply their knowledge and skills to the care of the population in need*

This relationship is only one of many that are crucial for population medicine if it is to deliver on the Triple Aim. Healthcare professionals need to be able to work with social workers, teachers, police, and many others.

Ways in which value for the population in need can be maximised by hospital specialists working in partnership with generalists are shown in Display 1.3. It is important to emphasise that the specialist or consultant with responsibility for a population does not become responsible for every patient. The generalist (family doctor, primary care physician or general practitioner) retains responsibility for the patients who are registered with them, and the specialist does not become responsible for the clinical care of all the individuals in a population. Specialists, however, do become responsible for the health of all the people who have the condition about which they have specialist knowledge, and all the people who might develop it (i.e. those who are or could be in need). Thus, they are also

1. 很多全科医生和专科医生都未能理解症状、体征或检测结果的灵敏度与其阳性预测值之间的区别。在全科诊疗中，就诊人员的发病率和患病率较低。其症状、体征或阳性检测结果的影响要比在专科诊疗中小得多；全科医生通常将那些明显患病或患病概率更高的人转诊给专科医生。因此，专科就诊人员的发病率和患病率更高。所以，全科医生对症状、体征或检测结果的关注度远低于专科医生。这种情况导致专科医生经常批评全科医生漏诊那些"显而易见"的诊断，而全科医生则抱怨专科医生对患者过度检查。

2. 医疗问题的复合性（complex）和复杂性（complicated）是两个不同的概念。这里举例说明医疗问题的复合性：一位 80 岁的老太太，患有 4 种疾病且需要接受 7 种处方治疗，由自己 50 岁的女儿照料；而她 50 岁的女儿又有一个酗酒的丈夫和一个无业的儿子。这种情况在全科医生工作中很常见。当某种已被确诊的疾病恶化时，就出现了问题的复杂性，如一个帕金森患者出现了心力衰竭，此时全科医生就需要寻求专科医生的帮助。

为了实现医疗卫生保健对人群价值的最大化，重要的是：

- 帮助全科医生和专科医生通力合作；
- 认识到专科医生的知识和技能不仅要用于被转诊来的患者，也要用于没有被转诊来的患者；
- 鼓励并资助专科医生利用自己的知识和技能服务于有需求的人群。

群医学要实现三重目标（Triple Aim）[①]，全科医生和专科医生之间的关系只是应当理顺的各项关键之一。医疗卫生保健专业人员需要与社会工作者、教师、警察和其他各界人士合作。

场景 1.3 展示了全科医生和专科医生合作以最大限度地满足人群需求的方法。需要强调的是，对人群负责的专科或主任医师并不意味着需要对每一个患者负责。通科医生（家庭医生、初级卫生保健医生或全科医生）仍需要对在他们名下登记在册的患者负责，而专科医生不需要对人群中每个个体的临床护理负责。然而，由于专科医生掌握了某种疾病的专业知识，他们也的确需要对所有患有这种疾病的人以及将来可能患这种疾病的人（即那些需要

---

① 三重目标的含义可参见序言脚注。

responsible not just for the quality and value of care delivered for people with the relevant condition, but also for the prevention of that condition and for helping people with that condition lead a full and healthy life.

Display 1.3 Specialists and generalists working in partnership to take a population approach to chronic obstructive pulmonary disease (COPD)

Scenario: A specialist service for COPD at which 800 patients a year are seen by the consultant in respiratory medicine

- Specialist service to estimate the number of patients with COPD in the population covered by the clinical networks in which the consultant works, based on published epidemiological studies and prescribing data (~ 2000)
- Conduct an audit across the clinical networks to identify people who have not been referred but who would benefit from referral (~ 200)
- Hold a joint discussion about how to increase productivity: whether the specialist service should see 1000 extra patients a year using the same level of resources or whether general practitioners (GPs) manage 200 of the 800 people referred if the GPs are given more support by the specialist service
- Specialist service to identify, through an analysis of prescribing and referral patterns, the scope for the specialist service to give greater support to certain GPs
- Specialist service to ensure that important new evidence reaches all those healthcare professionals who need to be aware of it
- Specialist service to ensure that all people with COPD receive unbiased information
- Specialist service to accept responsibility for the local variant of the Map of Medicine®
- Specialist service to take responsibility for the professional development of all GPs, physiotherapists and pharmacists who are seeing patients with COPD in the population covered by the network
- Specialist service to coordinate and lead the network of all relevant professionals and patient organisations
- Specialist service to produce an annual report

To enable clinicians to fulfil all the responsibilities of population medicine:
- *these responsibilities need to be recognised in clinicians' job descriptions*
- *time should be allocated to enable clinicians to carry out these responsibilities*

The lead consultant, however, may also require support for the coordination of the network, with help from a clinical scientist or administrator. A job description with key responsibilities for the clinician who takes the leading role for population medicine is set out in Display 1.4, although it is not envisaged that many clinicians will be engaged full-time in population medicine.

或可能需要帮助的人）的健康负责。因此，他们不仅要为相关疾病患者提供质量合格的医疗卫生保健服务，还要负责预防此类疾病发生，并帮助患者安享充实健康的生活。

场景 1.3　全科医生和专科医生合作，以群医学工作方式应对慢性阻塞性肺疾病

情况：一项专科服务，每年由呼吸科主任医生为 800 名慢性阻塞性肺疾病（慢阻肺）患者看诊

- 专科医生利用临床工作网络中的流行病学研究和处方数据，对他们服务的人群中慢阻肺患者的数量进行估算（约 2000）
- 在临床网络上审核复查那些没有转诊至专科医生、但可以通过转诊获益的患者（约 200）
- 全科医生与专科医生一同讨论如何提高服务效率：在使用同样的卫生资源情况下，专科医生在一年内是否有能力多服务 1000 名患者；或全科医生在专科医生更多的帮助下，是否能仅转诊 800 名患者中的 200 名
- 通过对处方和转诊模式展开分析，确定专科医生可以在多大程度上给予某些全科医生以更大的支持
- 专科医生需确保那些有必要知晓最新循证信息的医疗卫生保健专业人员能够获得这些信息
- 专科医生需要确保所有慢阻肺患者获得准确无误的信息
- 当医疗片区的划分有变动时，专科医生承担相应的职责
- 专科医生应该帮助全科医生、物理治疗师和药剂师提高专业素质，以服务那些工作网络覆盖人群中的慢阻肺患者
- 专科医生需要协调和领导工作网络内所有的专业组织和患者团体
- 此项专科服务每年生成一份年度报告

为了让临床医生能够履行群医学的全部职责：

- 这些职责需要在临床医生的岗位描述中得到明确；
- 需要给临床医生一定的时间以履行这些职责。

然而，主管的专科医生可能仍要行政人员和临床科研人员协助开展工作网络。场景 1.4 列举了主管群医学工作的临床医生的岗位描述和主要职责，但这并不意味着很多临床医生将全职从事群医学工作。

Display 1.4 Job description for a lead clinician with responsibility for population medicine, taking neurological disease as an example

Aim	To improve the health of all the people with neurological disease in the local population served
Key result areas	To promote the prevention of neurological disease To develop and maintain estimates of the total numbers of people with common neurological disease and problems For each common neurological disease, to ensure that there is a system of care with appropriate criteria and standards, and that each system is expressed as a care pathway To build and sustain a clinical network To work with patients and their representatives to help people with neurological disease to participate as partners in their care and to live a full life and to have a good death To promote research To produce an annual report for the population served
Resources	The post-holder will have one day a week reserved for this work. They will be supported by an information scientist with knowledge management skills working two days a week and have a small budget to facilitate their work
Key relationships	Local branches of relevant patient groups Local branches of relevant professional associations Public health professionals serving the population Relevant managers and policy-makers

■ The ethical issues of population medicine

When the topic of population medicine is first raised, some clinicians will be concerned about a potential ethical conflict, as they perceive it, between their commitment to the individual patient and an explicit responsibility to the population. In reality, clinicians have always had to manage that most precious of resources, their time, not only by considering what the patient in front of them wants but also the needs of other patients.

In situations where clinicians have to make judgements about whether to allocate additional financial resources to the patient in front of them, this does present an ethical problem. This problem can be prevented by ensuring that decisions about the allocation of resources are not made by an individual clinician during a consultation, but through a process that is open and accountable.

At the beginning of the 21st century, an increasing number of people would agree that it is now unethical not to consider the whole population as well as the individual patient. The principal argument in the debate is about environmental change and resource use, as opposed to lower-value healthcare. These environmental issues, however, are highly relevant and relate to the phenomenon known as 'the

场景 1.4　主管群医学的临床医生岗位描述——以神经医学为例

目标	•提高服务地区人群神经系统疾病患者的健康水平
达成的关键结果	•促进神经系统疾病的预防 •定期评估该地区常见神经系统疾病的患病人数 •为每一种常见的神经系统疾病建立卫生保健体系，包括适宜的标准和规范，每一体系都以工作路径展现 •建立并维持临床工作网络 •与患者及其代理人合作，帮助神经系统疾病患者参与自身护理，过上充实生活、安详离世 •推动相关研究 •为服务人群提供一份年度报告
资源	•负责该岗位的医生每周预留一天时间从事本项（群医学）工作。那些具有知识管理技能的信息学专家则每周用两天时间为其提供帮助，也需要一点资金以支持他们开展工作
核心关系	•相关患者组织在当地的分支机构 •相关专业协会在地方的分支机构 •为人群服务的公共卫生专业人员 •相关管理人员和政策制定者

■ 群医学的伦理问题

群医学首次被提出时，一些临床医生担心：在他们对个体患者的承诺和对人群的明确责任之间存在潜在的伦理冲突。实际上，临床医生总是不得不管理他们最宝贵的资源——时间，他们不仅要考虑他们面前的患者需要什么，还要考虑其他患者的需求。

在临床医生必须判断是否应该为面前患者分配额外的财政资源时，确实面临伦理问题。要想避免这一问题，就需要确保资源配置决策过程是公开和可信的，而不是由某个临床医生在提供就诊咨询服务期间擅自决定。

21世纪初，越来越多的人认为，对全部人群和对个体患者的忽视都是不符合伦理的。这场争论主要论点在于环境的变化和资源的利用，而非低质量的医疗卫生保健。然而，这些环境问题都与"公地的悲剧"[①]密切相关，在

---

① 指涉及个人利益与公共利益对稀缺资源分配有所冲突的社会陷阱。

tragedy of the commons' in which environmental degradation occurs whenever many individuals use a scarce resource in common (see Display 1.5). Reuben argues that this is the situation in healthcare (3). If every clinician and every patient uses more and more of the finite healthcare resources, there will come a point when the health service breaks down and everyone suffers.

Display 1.5 The tragedy of the commons (4)

Scenario: Imagine you are a farmer grazing your sheep on common land
Custom and tradition mean that you are allowed to have 20 sheep on the common land, but you introduce one more and no-one seems to notice or mind. So the next year you introduce another sheep, and the following year another, and so on. Unfortunately, all the other commoners have done the same thing such that a point is reached when the whole ecosystem collapses, the grass does not grow and all the sheep die. This is the tragedy of the commons.

Apart from the danger of service breakdown, in healthcare the balance between benefit and harm changes with the increasing investment of resources: benefit is subject to the law of diminishing returns, whereas harm increases in direct proportion to the resources invested. Indeed, a point may be reached when the increased investment of resources will lead to a reduction in net benefit. Thus, it is important to be cautious about using increased resources, not simply from a financial perspective but also from the perspective of maximising the balance of benefit to harm for the population served.

During the 20th century, healthcare professionals provided health services on the assumption that 'more is better'; however, there is a new paradigm for the 21st century:

In medicine there are three do's; the can do, the actually do and the should do ... with the aging of the population and the proliferation of the can do, the increase in future healthcare capabilities and costs is an impending tragedy of the commons. The most important challenge for the 21st century is not to expand the can do; rather, it is to bring the care that is provided into line with the should do. Failure to do so will result in a healthcare system that will certainly be fiscally, if not morally, bankrupt. (3)

Reuben makes an important point here. Too often, we confuse exhaustiveness-the tendency to leave no stone unturned – with appropriateness and optimality.

■ New skills for population medicine

This book, Population Medicine, has been prepared to help the general practitioner consortia and hospital and mental health specialists, both medical

这一"悲剧"中，每当许多人使用一种共同的稀缺资源时，就会发生环境的退化（场景 1.5）。鲁本认为：这就是医疗面临的实际情况[3]。如果每个临床医生和每个患者都越来越多地使用有限的医疗资源时，卫生资源总有一天会崩溃，而每个人也都会遭殃。

场景 1.5　公地的悲剧[4]

情况：假如你是一个在公共土地上放羊的农民
按照习惯和传统，只允许你在公共土地上养 20 只羊，但你多养了一只，似乎没有人注意或介意。第二年你又多养了一只，第三年你又多养一只，以此类推。不幸的是，所有农民都采取了相同策略，直至到达临界点，然后整个生态系统崩溃，草不再生长，所有的羊都死了，这就是公地的悲剧。

除了崩溃的危险，还需要意识到，在医疗卫生保健中随着投资的增加，损益平衡会发生变化：投资收益遵从收益递减规律，而投资风险则随着投资增多而增加。的确，当投资增多到达临界点后，增加资源投入所带来的净收益会逐渐减少。因此，谨慎使用已增加的资源非常重要，不仅要从财务角度，还要从为所服务的人群获取最大利益的角度来考虑。

在 20 世纪，医疗卫生专业人员是基于"越多越好"的理念来提供医疗卫生保健服务的，然而在 21 世纪，出现了新的范式：

> 　　卫生服务有"三做"——能做、实做、该做。随着人口老龄化，以及"能做"的激增，未来医疗服务的能力和成本的增加将是一个迫在眉睫的"公地的悲剧"。21 世纪最大的挑战不是扩充"能做"，相反，应当是我们所提供的卫生保健服务应以"该做"为原则。如果做不到这一点，我们的医疗卫生保健服务体系一定会出现崩溃——不在财政上就在道德上[3]。

鲁本在这里提出了一个重要的观点：我们常常把耗尽性（exhaustiveness，用尽一切手段的倾向）和最适性（appropriateness）、最佳性（optimality）混为一谈。

■ 群医学的新技能

《群医学》这本书将会帮助全科医生及医院、精神卫生专家（医学或非

and non-medical, to develop the knowledge and skills they need for the task of practising and delivering population medicine. It is focused primarily on the new responsibilities of clinicians, and in particular their responsibility to the whole population, rather than just their responsibility to the proportion of the population in contact with the service. As previously outlined, for acute, unequivocal health needs, such as a broken leg, the whole population in need accesses the right service, but this is not the case for many people with chronic health problems.

The skills for population medicine complement and supplement the skills that many clinicians have acquired during the last two decades. Although this new skill set includes general management skills and techniques to improve quality and safety, the skills necessary to maximise value for the whole population, as well as to improve quality and safety for individual patients, have not hitherto been covered. See Box 1.1.

Box 1.1 The skills for population medicine

- Maximising value
- Reducing waste and increasing sustainability
- Mitigating inequity
- Promoting health and preventing disease
- Creating systems
- Building networks
- Clarifying pathways
- Developing budgets
- Managing knowledge
- Engaging the population and patients
- Changing the culture

■ Questions for reflection

- *What are the ethical issues for clinicians whose only concern is for the patients who consult them?*
- *If we accept that responsibility for quality, equity and ensuring patients are treated with dignity are all essential aspects of good healthcare, are there any other responsibilities in addition to the seven listed which clinicians need to fulfil in the 21st century?*
- *Why should all clinicians be explicitly responsible for some or all of the seven new responsibilities?*

医学的）掌握必要的知识和技能，以使他们能够承担和开展群医学工作。这本书首要关注的是临床医生的新责任，特别是他们对整个人群的责任，而不仅仅是对那些已接触到医疗的人们负责。如前所述，对那些急性的、需求明确的疾病如腿部骨折，有医疗需求的人皆可以获得妥善处治，但这对许多有慢性疾病的患者来说，情况却不然。

群医学的技能是对很多临床医生在过去 20 年获得的工作技能的补充和完善。尽管这套新技能包含了那些可以提高质量及安全性的一般的管理技能和技术。但是迄今为止，如何使医疗卫生保健对于全人群的价值最大化以及如何提高对个体患者的服务质量及安全性，临床医生依旧欠缺这些方面所需的技能。这就是群医学所需要解决的问题（专栏 1.1）。

专栏 1.1 群医学的新技能

- 将价值最大化
- 减少资源浪费，提高可持续性
- 减少不平等
- 促进健康和预防疾病
- 构建体系
- 建立工作网络
- 理清工作路径
- 制定预算
- 管理知识
- 动员民众和患者
- 改变文化

■ 思考题

- 如果临床医生只关注前来咨询就诊的患者，这将面临怎样的伦理问题？
- 如果我们认同确保医疗服务的质量、公平及患者在诊疗中得到尊重，这些职责都是好的医疗卫生实践的不可或缺的方面，那么除了本章提到的 21 世纪临床医生应当履行的 7 项职责外，还有哪些职责？
- 为什么所有的临床医生都应该明确地承担对本章提到的 7 项责任中的一部分或全部？

── References ──────────────────────────────────────

Population medicine – accountability to and for a population

(1) Mitton C, Donaldson C. Priority setting toolkit: A guide to the use of economics in healthcare decision making. BMJ 2004: 5–6.

(2) Block P. Stewardship: choosing service over self-interest. California: Barrett-Koehler; 1996.

— 参 考 文 献 —

The ethical issues of population medicine

(3) Reuben D. Miracles, choices and justice: the tragedy of the future commons. JAMA 2010; 304: 467–468.

(4) Ostrom E. Governing the Commons: The Evolution of Institutions for Collective Action. Cambridge: Cambridge University Press; 1990.

1.2 Towards population health

In this section, we explore:

• *moving from a paradigm of institutions to systems*

• *why every health service must play a part in disease prevention*

• *how to explain the term 'equity', and in what ways it differs from equality*

• *how to explore the issue of equity, the Inverse Care Law and unmet need in your service at the population level*

■ From great institutions to great systems

In the Middle Ages, people built cathedrals; in the 19th century, they built railway stations; in the 20th century, they built hospitals. Many hospitals are huge, sprawling sites, continually evolving and never reaching completion.

Hospitals became the sites for the delivery of specialist services, and also sites for the development of super-specialist services; these services came to be called secondary and tertiary care, respectively. Mental health services developed in the 19th century, and often took the form of asylums located on the edge of towns and cities remote from the hospitals, even though many of the residents had physical as well as mental health problems, as is the case today.

In the second half of the 20th century, two new institutions developed – general practice and government-run community services. General practice evolved from being composed of isolated practitioners in private practice to being a powerful collegial force. Community services replaced the voluntary and charitable services that had cared for the elderly, the infirm and children.

In numerous national settings, healthcare is an archipelago of institutions, with four great islands connected by the occasional ferry (Figure 1.9).

第 2 节 人群健康

在本节中，我们将探讨：

- 从机构范式转向系统范式；

- 为什么每种医疗卫生保健服务都必须在疾病预防中发挥作用；

- 如何解释"公平"一词，它与"平等"的不同之处；

- 如何从人群层面来探讨公平、医疗逆向照护法则和医疗服务中未满足的需求等问题。

■ 从大机构到大系统

中世纪的人们建造大教堂；19 世纪的人们建造火车站；20 世纪的人们则忙着建造医院。许多医院都是杂乱无章的庞然大物，不断扩张，从未竣工。

医院成为提供专科医疗的场所，亚专科也在此处蜕变而出——这分别被称为二级和三级医疗卫生保健服务。19 世纪发展起来的精神卫生服务通常以收容所的形式运行，并且远离医院，位于城镇边缘[①]。尽管很多精神病患者同时也有躯体上的疾患，但仍在精神卫生服务场所接受治疗。时至今日，依然如此。

20 世纪后半叶出现了两类新型机构——全科诊疗机构和政府运行的社区服务机构。全科医生队伍由私营诊所中的一个个独立执业医生组成，逐渐发展壮大；而社区服务机构则取代了照顾年老体弱者和儿童的志愿服务和慈善服务。

在许多国家中，医疗卫生保健体系是由四个"孤岛"组成的，四大岛通过临时渡轮[②]相连（图 1.9）。

---

① 精神卫生服务独立于医疗卫生保健服务。
② 即转诊服务。

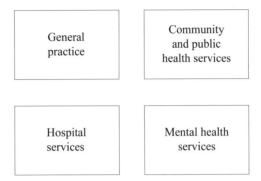

Figure 1.9   The healthcare archipelago

By the end of the 20th century, there was growing concern about the need to develop an integrated approach to common health problems through defining systems of care. (1) The exemplar of an integrated system of care is that for people with cancer. Faced with the considerable capital expense of providing radiotherapy, the managers of most district general hospitals accepted that investment in radiotherapy should take place in teaching hospitals. This intensity of investment at some but not all healthcare sites led to the creation of cancer networks, across which were delivered a system of care ranging from screening to end-of-life care. Constraints on capital investment also led to the development of systems for:

• *end-stage renal failure*

• *acute stroke*

• *myocardial infarction*

In a population-based system, the archipelago of care is transformed into a set of inter-related types of care which recognises that self-care is the most important (Figure 1.7).

Each system of care needs to have a focus. The various types of system focus for health services in countries with developed economies are shown in Box 1.2.

Box 1.2 The various types of focus for systems of care

• Symptoms or clinical presentations, such as breathlessness or back pain
• Diseases or conditions, such as inflammatory bowel disease, asthma or depression
• Subgroups of the population, such as frail elderly people or people under 65 years of age with multiple morbidities

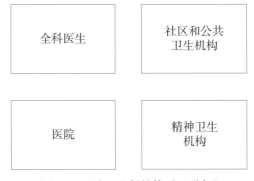

图 1.9　医疗卫生保健体系"群岛"

　　到了 20 世纪末，人们越来越觉得需要定义医疗卫生保健体系，建立整合型系统以应对普遍存在的健康问题[1]。一个整合型医疗系统的范例是为癌症患者提供的医疗卫生保健。由于提供放射治疗需要大量资金支持，大多数地区综合医院的管理者都认为仅应为教学医院的放射治疗投入资金。投资集中向少数机构促进了一些医疗机构（但并非所有）建立了癌症工作网络，并通过此类网络为患者提供从筛查到临终关怀的一系列服务。与癌症一样，经费短缺也促进了以下网络体系建立：

- 终末期肾功能衰竭；

- 急性卒中；

- 心肌梗死。

　　在一个以人群为基础的体系中，医疗卫生保健服务"群岛"会被转变为彼此密切关联的各种医疗服务，并把患者的自我照护看成是最重要的内容（图 1.7）。

　　每个医疗卫生保健体系都需要有一个关注点。专栏 1.2 展示了发达国家中医疗卫生保健服务系统的不同类型关注点。

专栏 1.2　医疗卫生保健体系中不同类型的关注点

- 症状或临床表现，如呼吸困难或背痛；

- 疾病或患病状况，如炎性肠病、哮喘或抑郁症；

- 人群中的亚人群，如年老体弱者或 65 岁以下有多种疾病的人。

There can be tension between generalists and specialists, but it is possible to minimise any tension by being clear about the relationship between complex and complicated health problems.

When discussing a condition such as asthma or epilepsy, it is common for general practitioners to point out that many of their patients have more than one problem. Indeed, people with multiple morbidities, often physical, mental and social, have complex problems – for example, an 84-year-old woman with four diagnoses and seven prescriptions being supported by a 50-year-old daughter with depression and a husband with an alcohol abuse problem. This is a complex problem but it is common in general practice. When one of the older woman's four problems, heart failure, for example, becomes complicated, the generalist needs to seek specialist advice. This highlights the relationship between complex and complicated problems, between the roles of generalist and specialist.

By contrast, in low- and middle-income countries, there is a move to create integrated primary care due to the inefficiencies that result from a collection of disease-based systems, such as onchocerciasis or malaria, which operate in isolation.

The development of systems of care does not reduce the need for good management of healthcare institutions, but it does require the skill to create and manage what have been called hybrid organisations, defined as organisations in which:

> ... functional units and mission orientated units work together and the accompanying principle of dual reporting, like a democracy, are not great in and of themselves. They just happen to be the best way for any business to be organised. (2)

Other people call this arrangement 'matrix management', the pattern for which is emerging in many countries (see Matrix 1.1).

Matrix 1.1 Matrix management

SYSTEMS							
FACILITIES		Cancer	Respiratory	Mental Health	Stroke	Frail Elderly	Children
	HR						
	Transport						
	Finance						
	Real Estate						
	IT						

全科医生和专科医生之间的关系可能会因为分歧变得紧张，但双方如果能清楚地了解健康问题的复合性（complex）和病情的复杂性（complicated）之间的关系，紧张关系就可以大大缓解。

当讨论哮喘或癫痫等疾病时，全科医生通常会指出，许多患者的问题都不止一种。事实上，患有多种障碍（常为生理、心理和社会方面等问题）的人，都有复合性问题——例如，一位患有 4 种确诊疾病，接受 7 种处方治疗的 84 岁妇女，正由 50 岁患有抑郁症且丈夫酗酒的女儿赡养，这就是诊疗中常见的复合性问题。当这位老年妇女的 4 种疾病之一——如心力衰竭——变得复杂时，全科医生需要寻求专科医生的建议。这强调了疾病的复合性和复杂性之间的关系就是全科医生和专科医生之间的关系。

相比之下，在低收入和中等收入国家，基于病种的（如盘尾丝虫病或疟疾）的医疗系统各自为政、效率低下，这些国家正在探索建立综合型初级医疗卫生保健体系。

医疗卫生保健体系的发展不仅要求医疗保健机构能够一如既往地良性管理，而且要求其具备建立和管理混合型组织的技能，即：

> ……一般职能部门和专业职能部门共事，以及随之而来的双重报告原则，就像民主制度，其自身及内在并不优越，但在组织任何事务时它们却正好是最佳方式[2]。

这种布局被称为"矩阵式管理"，此模式正出现在许多国家中（矩阵 1.1）。

矩阵 1.1　矩阵式管理

机构		系统					
		癌症	呼吸道疾病	精神卫生	卒中	年长体弱者	儿童
	人力资源						
	运输						
	财政						
	不动产						
	信息技术						

Andy Grove, who developed the definition of a hybrid organisation, was the Chief Executive of Intel and could control both dimensions of the matrix. The situation is more complex in healthcare where the contributions of different autonomous organisations must be integrated.

This challenge of complexity amplifies the need for the careful design of our systems of care (which we will explore in section 2.1), the development of appropriate networks to best deliver those systems (which we will explore in section 2.2), and the development of a supporting culture (which we will explore in section 2.3).

■ Promoting health and preventing disease

The meanings of 'health'

The meaning of the term 'health' is problematic and under continuous evolution. There is a general consensus, however, that a health service in isolation cannot promote health and prevent disease because it has no operational jurisdiction over almost all of the social determinants of health. Although all clinicians have a responsibility to promote health and prevent disease by providing information and support to the individual patients who consult them, this responsibility is of equal or greater significance for the clinician practising population medicine.

The well-known definition of health enshrined in the WHO Constitution of 1948 serves a useful function:

> *Health is a complete state of physical, mental and social well-being and not merely the absence of disease or infirmity. (3)*

Some authorities argue that this definition is too narrow. For Amartya Sen, the concept of health should encompass two further concepts:

- *social justice*
- *the societal responsibility to ensure that every individual has the capability of achieving their full potential (4)*

From Sen's perspective, health workers should be concerned about social injustice even if it does not cause disease or complicate treatment. Others, such as the distinguished philosopher Norman Daniels, suggest that health workers should focus on injustice and inequity only when they are complicating factors in the prevention or treatment of disease.

The clinician's contribution

In some countries, public health professionals view public health as a medical specialty. In other countries, in addition to the organisation of primary and

英特尔的首席执行官安迪·葛洛夫提出了混合型组织的概念，可控制矩阵的两个维度。在医疗卫生保健领域，情况更为复杂：必须整合不同自治组织在系统中所起作用。

这种复杂性的挑战进一步强调：有必要对医疗卫生保健体系进行精心设计（我们将在第 2 章第 1 节中探讨）及开发各种适用于这些系统的工作网络（我们将在第 2 章第 2 节中探讨），并发展相应的支持文化（我们将在第 2 章第 3 节中探讨）。

■ 促进健康和预防疾病

"健康" 的含义

"健康" 一词的含义一直存在争议并不断演变。然而，人们普遍认为，孤立的医疗卫生保健服务不能有效地促进健康并预防疾病，因为它对涉及健康的几乎所有社会决定因素都没有实际管辖权。尽管所有临床医生都有责任向前来咨询的患者提供信息和支持，帮助他们促进健康、预防疾病；但对于从事群医学的医生来说，这一职责具有同等或更多的内涵。

1948 年《世界卫生组织宪章》中所载的众所周知的、具有实用性的 "健康" 定义为：

> 健康是身体、精神和社会福祉（well-being）完好的一种整体状态，而不仅仅是没有疾病或身体虚弱[3]。

一些权威人士认为这一定义过于狭隘。阿马蒂亚·森就认为健康的概念还应包括以下两个的概念：

- 社会公正（social justice）；
- 确保每个人都能充分发挥全部潜力的社会责任[4]。

森认为，卫生工作者应该关注社会不公平，即使它不会引发疾病或使治疗复杂化；其他学者——如著名哲学家诺曼·丹尼尔斯——则认为，只有当不公正和不公平等因素影响到疾病的预防或治疗时，卫生工作者才应该关注它们。

临床医生的贡献

在一些国家，公共卫生专业人员将公共卫生视为一门医学专业；在另一

secondary preventive services (e.g. smoking cessation and screening, respectively), public health professionals focus on environmental protection or interpret their role as one of advocacy for social change.

Indeed, clinicians primarily involved in diagnosis, treatment and care can also have a very important role to play in disease prevention. For example, a clinician practising population medicine in order to prevent disease can ensure that:

- *everyone with heart disease, and not just those referred, are receiving aspirin and other evidence-based measures to control risk factors for a recurrent heart attack*
- *every person with chronic lung and heart disease is receiving flu immunisation*
- *every individual with tuberculosis is supported during the course of therapy until they have been cured*
- *all the relatives of people diagnosed with familial hypercholesterolaemia are identified and invited for testing*

Preventive healthcare is the most sustainable type of healthcare, but it requires focus and coordination, not only by public health professionals but also by practitioners of population medicine. Although some hospitals are now appointing public health professionals, this does not reduce the need for clinicians to be responsible for, and take action to improve, the health of the whole population in need.

Authority, leadership and action

Clinicians with management responsibilities have bureaucratic authority within the institution at which they fulfil those responsibilities. Clinicians practising population medicine will have some bureaucratic authority, but to fulfil their responsibilities they will also have to employ other forms of authority:

- *sapiential authority, derived from their knowledge*
- *charismatic authority, derived from their leadership position*

Management is mainly a transactional process, whereas leadership should be transformational. Thus, a leader not only has to deliver results but also has to transform organisations that serve the population. Transformational leadership may require that a clinician responsible for population medicine tries to improve the prevention of disease through advocacy by:

- *visiting the local Member of Parliament (MP)*
- *seeking to influence directly national or international policy-making*
- *ensuring that the relevant professional organisation is fully engaged in debates and decisions that could reduce the risk of disease at the population level*

Hospitals as health services

Language creates the culture within which people make decisions and express various behaviours. The traditional bureaucratic division of health services and the

些国家，除了组织实施初级和二级预防（如戒烟和筛查）服务，公共卫生专业人员还聚焦于环境保护，或视自身角色为社会变革的倡导者。

的确，临床医生主要从事诊断、治疗和照护的工作，但他们在疾病预防方面也可以发挥非常重要的作用。例如，为预防疾病而从事群医学的临床医生可以确保：

- 每个心脏病患者，而不仅仅是转诊过来的患者，都接受阿司匹林和其他循证干预措施，以控制引起复发性心肌梗死的危险因素；
- 每个患有慢性肺病和心脏病的人都接受流感疫苗接种；
- 每个肺结核患者在治疗过程中都会得到支持，直至治愈；
- 要找到被诊断为家族性高胆固醇血症的人的所有亲属，并都进行胆固醇检测。

预防性卫生保健服务是最具有可持续性的医疗卫生保健工作，但它不仅需要公共卫生专业人员，也需要群医学实践者们的关注与合作。虽然现在一些医院任命公共卫生专业人员从事这方面工作，但临床医生需要为整体人群健康负责并为之采取行动，这方面的需求从未减少。

权威、领导力和行动

具有管理职责的临床医生在履职机构中拥有行政权威。从事群医学的临床医生也拥有一些行政权威，但为了充分履职，他们还必须使用其他形式的权威：

- 源于知识的智慧权威；
- 来自领导地位的魅力权威。

管理主要是事务性的过程，而领导力应该具有变革性。因此，一个领导者不仅要交付成果，还必须改造为民众服务的组织。变革型领导力可能要求负责群医学的临床医生尝试以下方式以提高预防疾病的能力：

- 拜访当地政要；
- 试图直接影响国家或国际的政策制定；
- 确保相关专业机构有充分机会参加与减少人群疾病风险相关内容的讨论和决策。

医院作为医疗卫生保健服务机构

语言创造了文化，人们在其中做出决策、展示不同行为。医疗卫生保健机构在传统行政划分以及用来描述这些机构的语言——如与医疗卫生保健相

language used to describe these services – 'hospital' and 'community' in relation to care, and the separate identification of 'mental health services' – creates the wrong culture, one in which the hospital is assumed to be outside the community and only in the healthcare and not the health business (see Figure 1.9).

Hospital services, however, can play a major role in improving the health of the populations they serve, and acting as a public health service.

'Public health' is another term that causes confusion because it is, in one sense, a description of a professional group. In another sense, it is the outcome of the efforts of everyone seeking to prevent, diagnose and treat disease and promote health. Some hospitals are now setting up public health departments which have public health professionals within them, an approach referred to as 'the health-promoting hospital'. These departments sometimes focus on ensuring that every person who comes into hospital as a patient receives help to stop smoking. Although such moves are welcome, it is important not to create the impression that it absolves every other department in the hospital from using their opportunities and influence to promote health and prevent disease. Every hospital department has the ability to influence the health of the population served:

- *the trauma team can campaign against knife crime*
- *the hepatology service can campaign against harmful and hazardous drinking*
- *the cardiology service can promote healthy, balanced diets and physical activity*

In addition, the hospital as a whole can contribute to improving the health of the population it serves. For instance, in South Auckland, Counties Manukau Health decided not to recruit more nurses and health workers from the Philippines or Thailand but instead to set up a Health Academy to inspire, with great success, young people from the Māori and Pacific communities to aspire to become health workers at their base hospital, Middlemore.

■ Ethics and equity

Distinguishing equity from equality

Many people are confused about the difference between the terms 'equality' and 'equity', but the meaning of the two is quite different. Equality is measured objectively; equity is a subjective judgement of fairness.

Thus, a service may be supplied unequally and still be equitable (fair), and a service may by supplied equally and be inequitable (unfair).

关的"医院"和"社区"以及对"精神卫生机构"的单独划分——都产生了错误的文化；其中之一是认为"医院"应该设在社区之外，它只在医疗卫生保健范畴之内行事，而不属于卫生事业（图 1.9）。

然而，医院服务可以在改善其服务人群的健康方面发挥主要作用，而且是作为公共卫生服务发挥作用。

"公共卫生"是另一个引起混淆的术语，因为在某种意义上，它是对一个卫生专业队伍的描述；从另一种意义上来说，它是每个人在预防、诊断和治疗疾病并促进健康方面所付出努力的结果。现在一些医院设立了公共卫生科室，其中雇有公共卫生专业人员，并被称为"健康促进医院"。这些科室有时会把工作重点放在帮助那些求助戒烟的就诊者。尽管此举受到了欢迎，但重要的是不要给人留下这样的印象，即：医院的其他部门就没有责任利用机会和影响力以促进健康并预防疾病。医院的每个科室都有能力影响其服务整体人群的健康水平：

- 创伤救治小组可以呼吁打击持刀犯罪；
- 肝病服务中心可以开展反对有害饮酒的运动；
- 心脏病服务中心可以开展促进健康、均衡饮食运动的相关工作。

此外，医院可以作为一个整体为改善其服务整体人群的健康状况做出贡献。例如，在南奥克兰，马努考郡卫生局（Counties Manukau Health）决定不从菲律宾或泰国招聘更多的护士和卫生工作者，而是建立一所卫生学校，激励来自 Maori 和 Pacific 社区的年轻人成为当地基层医院——米德莫尔医院——的医疗卫生工作者，这项行动获得了极大的成功。

■ 伦理和公平

区分公平（equity）与平等（equality）

许多人对"平等"和"公平"的区别感到困惑，但这两个词的含义确实有很大的不同。平等（equality）是能客观衡量的；而公平（equity）则是对公平性（fairness）的主观判断。

因此，提供某一项服务可能是不平等的，但仍然会是公平的（即公正的）；而提供另一项服务虽可能是平等的，但却是不公平的（即不公正的）。

Health inequalities, such as people in lower-income groups dying younger or having a higher prevalence of disease than those in higher-income groups, are measured and reported using criteria such as the standardised mortality ratio (SMR). In all countries, there is marked inequality among different social groups: the greater the level of deprivation, the higher the mortality rate. In New Zealand and Australia, this is borne out in the lower life-expectancy of indigenous populations. (5, 6)

The relationship between deprivation and ill-health is mediated through 'the social determinants of health', a term developed and popularised by Michael Marmot. (7)

Inequalities in health service provision, however, do not follow the same pattern as inequalities in health; it is obvious that the distribution of many health services bears no consistent relationship to levels of deprivation in populations. There can be marked variation for many aspects of health service provision among similarly wealthy populations and among similarly deprived populations.

It is vital that the clinician responsible for population medicine takes account of the health inequalities in the local population. This is important because as part of a strategy to improve the health of the whole population, it is necessary to try to reduce the level of health inequalities.

In fact, recent cross-national evidence suggests that the greater the degree of socio-economic inequality that exists within a society, the steeper the gradient of health inequality. As a result, middle-income groups in a more unequal society will have worse health than comparable or even poorer groups in a society with greater equality. (8)

Classifying inequity in health services

As described above, inequality is not the same as inequity. Thomas Rice, a highly respected economist, emphasises the importance of distinguishing between the concepts of equality and equity:

The former implies equal shares of something; the latter, a 'fair' or 'just' distribution, which may or may not result in equal shares. (9)

There are several different types of inequity in the provision of health services (see Box 1.3).

健康方面的不平等，如低收入群体比高收入群体的死亡年龄更小或患病率更高，是以标准化死亡率（SMR）作为衡量和报告的标准。在所有国家，不同社会群体之间存在明显的不平等：贫困程度越高，死亡率就越高。在新西兰和澳大利亚，土著居民的预期寿命较低就证明了这一点[5, 6]。

贫困和不健康之间的关系是由"健康问题社会决定因素"来分析判断的，该术语由迈克尔·马尔莫特提出并推广[7]。

然而，医疗卫生保健供给方面的不平等与健康方面的不平等并不遵循同样的模式；很明显，许多医疗卫生服务的分配与人口的贫困程度没有一致性。在同等富裕或贫穷的人口中，在提供医疗卫生保健许多方面都可能存在明显的差异。

负责群医学的临床医生必须考虑到在当地人口中存在的健康不平等。这一点很重要，因为作为改善全民健康战略的一部分，必须努力减少健康不平等的程度。

事实上，最近的多国证据表明，一个社会中存在的社会经济不平等程度越高，健康不平等的梯度就越大。因此，在一个更不平等的社会中，其中等收入群体的健康状况会劣于在一个更平等的社会中有同等收入甚至收入更低的群体[8]。

对医疗卫生保健服务中不公平的分类

如上所述，不平等并不等同于不公平。托马斯·赖斯（Thomas Rice）这位备受尊敬的经济学家，强调要区分平等（equality）和公平（equity）概念的重要性：

前者意味着对某东西享有同等份额；后者意指在分配上要"公正"（fair）或"正义（just）"，但在份额上则可能"会"或"不一定会"同等[9]。

在提供医疗卫生保健服务方面有几种类型的不公平（专栏 1.3）。

Box 1.3 Types of inequity in the provision of health services

• Age-related: when older people are denied treatment simply because of their age

• Gender-related: when women receive effective treatment less frequently than men (10)

• Ethnicity-related: when members of a particular ethnic group receive less care than members of other ethnic groups despite the same level of or greater need as a result of cultural insensitivity, racism or discrimination (11, 12)

• Social: when one socio-economic group, almost always the most deprived, does not have the same access to healthcare as other socio- economic groups

If there are lower rates of intervention in one subgroup of the population which has the same, or greater, need than the population as a whole, this would suggest there are problems with the equity of provision. If patients in one subgroup of the population receive treatment at a later stage in the course of the disease than patients in another subgroup, this would also suggest problems with the equity of provision. In a study of equity of access to total joint replacement of hip and knee in England, Judge et al. (13) concluded that people in affluent areas got most provision relative to need (see Figure 1.10).

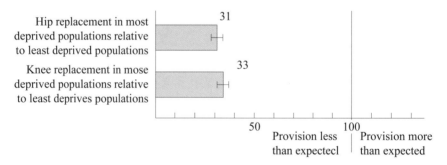

Figure 1.10   Inequities in the provision of hip and knee replacement (13)

It is also important to be aware that there can be situations in which inequality is equitable. For instance, a health service may decide to provide more resources to a deprived population because the need is greater than that in a less-deprived population.

Process equity should be the goal of health systems. There are several ways in which process equity can be defined.

• *Equal access to health care for equal need*

• *Equal use of health care for equal need*

• *Equal health care expenditure for equal need*

专栏 1.3　在提供医疗卫生保健服务方面，不公平（inequity）的类型

- 与年龄相关的不公平：老年人仅仅因为年龄过大而被拒绝给予治疗。
- 与性别有关的不公平：女性接受有效治疗的频率低于男性[10]。
- 与种族有关的不公平：某一族群对医疗卫生保健服务需求与其他族群相比相差无异或者更大，但由于文化钝感、种族主义或歧视，该族群成员得到的照顾少于其他族群成员[11, 12]。
- 源于社会性的不公平：当某一社会经济群体（几乎总是最贫困的群体），得不到其他社会经济群体同样的医疗卫生保健服务使用权时。

　　当一个亚人群具有与总人群相同的或更大的需求，但其得到的干预率水平却低于总人群，这就意味着在供给的公平性上存在着问题。如果相同疾病的患者仅因为所属的亚人群不同，接受治疗的时间就有所差异，这也是在供应的公平性方面存在问题。在英国进行髋膝关节置换术的公平性研究中，贾琦（Judge）等人得出的结论是，富裕地区的人们获得了最能满足需求的供给量（图 1.10）[13]。

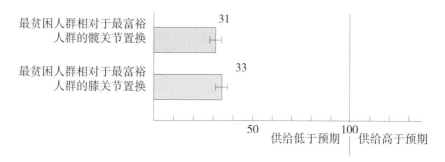

图 1.10　在髋膝关节置换术方面存在的供给不公平

　　在某些情况下，不平等（inequality）是公平的（equitable）。认识到这点同样重要。例如，卫生服务机构可能决定向贫困人群提供更多资源，因为这些人的需求大于那些相对富裕的人群。

　　程序公平应该是卫生体系的目标。通过以下方法可以定义程序公平：

- 需求相同者有同等获得医疗卫生服务的机会；
- 需求相同者使用了同等医疗卫生保健服务；
- 为需求相同者支付了同等医疗费用。

All of these refer to equity between people with the same health care needs. This is known as horizontal equity. It is also important to recognize the corollary, that people with different or unequal needs should receive different or unequal health care. This is known as vertical equity. (14)

Another dimension to the concept of healthcare inequity relates to the quality of care provided and not just the volume of care or activity levels. In 1971, Julian Tudor Hart, an exceptional general practitioner, published an article describing the Inverse Care Law, which states that:

The availability of good medical care tends to vary inversely with the need for it in the population served. (15)

A clear illustration of the Inverse Care Law in operation is the experience of single homeless people whose needs are high but who, in most cities, have very poor access to care and therefore receive less high-value care.

Identifying inequity

Some of the root causes of inequity are beyond the power of the medical profession to solve, but the individual clinician with responsibility for a population can mitigate the effects of inequity by identifying people within the population who are likely to be experiencing inequity (see Box 1.4).

Box 1.4 Ways to identify inequity in the population being served

- Compare the number of patients seen from different subgroups within the population, e.g. from different general practices, social groups, or ethnic groups
- Audit referrals to identify differences in levels of need at the point of referral in different groups of patients

Having identified inequity, the clinician responsible for a population can take action by:

- *making a direct approach to the relevant subgroups in the population*
- *visiting health centres serving populations from which referrals seem too few*

It is difficult, however, for any clinician to achieve much as an individual. It is important to persuade the healthcare organisation to take action:

所有这些都是指具有相同医疗卫生需求的人之间的公平。这就是所谓的横向公平。以此类推，需求不同或不平等的人在得到医疗卫生服务方面就也应该相应地不同或不平等。这就是所谓的纵向公平[14]。

医疗卫生不公平的另一个概念与其质量有关，而不仅只是服务的数量或频次。1971 年，朱利安·都铎·哈特，一位杰出的全科医生，发表了一篇关于逆向照护法则①的文章，文章指出：

在一个地区，高质量医疗保健的可获得性往往与所服务人群的需要成反比[15]。

单身流浪汉的经历清楚地说明了逆向照护法则是真实存在的。他们的卫生需求很高，但在大多数城市获得医疗卫生保健的机会很低，所得到的高质量医疗卫生服务也更少。

识别不公平

消除某些不公平的根源性因素非医学界力所能及，但负责群体健康的临床医生自己可以通过识别出人群中可能遭受不公平待遇的那些人，进而减轻不公平带来的影响（专栏 1.4）。

专栏 1.4　识别服务人群中不公平的方法

- 比较人群中来自不同亚组的患者数量，如来自不同的全科门诊、社会群体或种族群体；
- 审核转诊，以确定不同患者组在转诊点的需求水平上的差异。

在识别出不公平之后，负责该人群的临床医生可以采取以下措施：

- 直接接触人群中的相关亚人群组；
- 访问那些转诊人数过少的医疗卫生服务中心。

然而，作为个体，任何临床医生都很难取得很大成就。因此，说服医疗卫生保健机构采取措施是很重要的：

---

① 逆向照护法则（invese care law）是朱立安·哈特在 1971 年提出，是指越是需要医疗照护及社会关怀的人，其可得到的资源反而越少，考虑到医疗卫生保健实际内涵，本书译为"逆向照护法则"。

- *by including representatives of the most deprived subgroups in the population on boards and management groups*
- *by investing in the local population, through establishing scholarships at local schools and colleges with the aim of recruiting more local people into the healthcare professions and workforce*

At Ko Awatea and Counties Manukau Health, together with our academic partners, we have developed and resourced a career 'pipeline' to identify, support, and develop the future healthcare professionals from the community we serve. We cannot hope to transform the community in which we work unless our staff understand, reflect, and comprise our local community. In addition, a health worker in a family increases health literacy, increases income, and builds a virtuous cycle in which they become role models for future health professionals from their families and community.

Equity and social justice

Leaders of any healthcare organisation must appreciate the multidimensional nature of equity; as a concept, it cannot be understood solely in terms of the distribution of healthcare.

> *Health equity ... includes the fairness of processes and thus must attach importance to non-discrimination in the delivery of health care. Furthermore, an adequate engagement with health equity also requires that the considerations of health be integrated with broader issues of social justice and overall equity, paying adequate attention to the versatility of resources and the diverse reach and impact of different social arrangements. (4)*

Equity is a matter of social justice, and any publicly funded health service has a part to play in creating a just society as well as a healthy society. Indeed, some would argue that a population cannot be healthy if there is significant injustice.

> *Justice ... requires meeting health care needs fairly under resource constraints and this, in turn, requires limiting care in a publicly accountable way. (16)*

Taking this perspective, health promotion encompasses efforts not only to change individuals' lifestyles but also to promote social justice.

- 将人群中最贫困群体的代表纳入管理委员会或管理小组；
- 通过向当地人群投资，在当地学校和大学设立奖学金，目的是吸引更多的当地年轻人加入医疗卫生保健服务行业。

在寇·阿瓦提中心（Ko Awatea）[①] 和马努考郡卫生局，我们与学术合作伙伴一起建立并投资了一个"定向卫生保健人员培养项目"，目的是为所服务社区发现、支持并培养未来的医疗专业人员。除非我们自己能理解、反思并成为当地社区一员，否则不能奢望我们所工作的社区会被改造。此外，一个医疗卫生工作者在自己家庭内应该提高健康素养，增加收入，并建立良性循环——在循环中，他们将成为家庭和社区未来医疗专业人员的榜样。

公平和社会正义

任何医疗卫生保健组织的领导者都必须认识到公平的多维性；公平作为一个概念，不能仅仅从医疗卫生分配上来理解。

> 健康的公平……包括程序公平，因此在提供医疗卫生保健时，必须重视非歧视原则。此外，充分实施健康方面的公平，还需要把健康方面的考虑因素与社会公正和总体公平等更广泛的问题相结合；也要充分注意资源的灵活性以及不同社会安排的范围和多种影响[(4)]。

公平反映的是一种社会正义。任何公共资助的医疗服务应对创建健康和公正的社会发挥作用。当然有些人还会争论说，如果存在严重的社会不公正现象，那么人群就不可能健康。

> 公正……需要在资源有限时、公平地满足医疗卫生保健的需求。反过来，也需要以对公众负责的方式、对医疗卫生保健服务的范围有所限制[(16)]。

从这个角度来看，促进健康不仅应包括改变个人生活方式的努力，还应致力于促进社会的公正。

---

① 此为马努考郡卫生局的卫生系统创新和改进研究所。

■ Questions for reflection

- *What can be done by any health service to tackle inequity in access to healthcare when the causes of inequity are so deeply embedded in society?*
- *When considering your service, which subgroups in the local population are at greatest risk of inequity?*
- *What could you do next year to reduce inequity in your service?*

References

From great institutions to great systems

(1) Gray JAM. Four Box Healthcare: Planning in a Time of Zero Growth. Lancet. 1983; 2: 1185–1186.

(2) Grove AS. High Output Management. New York: Vintage Books; 1995. Promoting health and preventing disease

(3)World Health Organization (WHO) Preamble to the Constitution of the World Health Organization as adopted by the International Health Conference, New York, 19 June–22 July 1946; signed on 22 July 1946 by the representatives of 61 States (Official Records of the World Health Organization, no. 2, p. 100) and entered into force on 7 April 1948. Website http://www.who.int/suggestions/faq/en/index.html.Accessed 14 July 2014.

(4) Sen A. Why Health Equity? In: Anand S, Peter F, Sen A, Eds. Public Health, Ethics, and Equity. Oxford: Oxford University Press; 2004.

Ethics and equity

(5) Demographic Trends: 2011. Statistics New Zealand Website. www.stats.govt.nz. Accessed July 2014.

(6) The Health and Welfare of Australia's Aboriginal and Torres Strait Islander Peoples. Australian Bureau of Statistics Website. www.abs.gov.au. Accessed July 2014.

(7) Closing the gap in a generation: Health equity through action on the social determinants of health; report of the Commission chaired by Michael Marmot. World Health Organization; 2008.

■ 思考题

• 当不平等的成因深深地根植于社会之中时，每个医疗卫生服务机构都可以做些什么来解决医疗卫生方面的不平等问题？

• 谈及您所提供的医疗卫生保健服务，当地人群中的哪一个亚群体可能面临最大的不公平风险？

• 在您的医疗卫生保健项目中，明年您打算做些什么来减少其中的不公平？

参 考 文 献

(8) Daniels N, Kennedy B, Kawachi I. Health and Inequality, or, Why Justice is Good for Our Health. In: Anand S, Peter F, Sen A, Eds. Public Health, Ethics, and Equity. Oxford: Oxford University Press; 2004: 63.

(9) Rice T. The Economics of Health Reconsidered. Baltimore: Health Administration Press; 1998: 152.

(10) Alspach JG. Is there gender bias in critical care? Critical Care Nurse. Dec 2012; 32: 8-14.

(11) Pamuk E, Mukuc D, Heck K, Reuben C, Lochner K. Socioeconomic status and health chartbook. Health, United States, 1998. Hyattsville, Maryland: National Center for Health Statistics; 1998.

(12) Crimmins EM, Kim JK, Alley DE, Karlamangla A, Seeman T. Hispanic paradox in biological risk profiles. American Journal of Public Health. Jul 2007; 97: 1305-10.

(13) Judge A et al. (2010) Equity in access to total joint replacement of hip and knee in England. BMJ. 2010; 341: 4092.

(14) Wonderling D, Gruen R, Black N. Introduction to Health Economics: Understanding Public Health. Maidenhead: Open University Press; 2005: 157.

(15) Hart JT. The Inverse Care Law. Lancet. 1971; 392: 48–49.

(16) Daniels N, Sabin J. Setting Limits Fairly. Learning to share resources for health. 2nd Edition. Oxford: Oxford University Press; 2008: 3.

1.3 Towards patient experience

In this section, we explore:
- *obtaining the right outcome for each individual patient*
- *engaging patients and populations*
- *the importance of patient engagement in health service development and delivery*
- *how engagement can improve the quality and increase the value of healthcare*
- *how patient engagement can inform the debate about resource allocation and resource constraints*
- *the importance and dual role of patients' organisations*

■ Getting the right outcome for each individual patient

Changing the traditional view of the 'right' patient outcome

For decades, the definition of 'right' was established by medical opinion until Archie Cochrane published his book Effectiveness and Efficiency in 1972. (1) The application of Cochrane's principles to clinical practice was first called 'clinical epidemiology'. (2) Subsequently, the concept of evidence-based medicine has been developed (3), which emphasises that the making of clinical decisions should be based on best current evidence and not established medical opinion.

Evidence-based medicine (EBM) requires the integration of the best research evidence with our clinical expertise and our patient's unique values and circumstances. (3)

Personalising decisions

The 'right' thing for individual patients is determined by the decisions made by clinicians and patients. For every million population, many decisions are made in the 40,000 consultations that take place daily. These decisions may be shared between clinicians and patients to a greater or lesser degree during a consultation, but many are taken by either clinicians or patients outside the consultation, such as a patient's decision not to take the medication prescribed for them. The total number of decisions daily is difficult to estimate, but it could be more than 200,000 per million population. These decisions influence both patient outcomes and cost.

第 3 节　患者体验

在本节中，我们将探讨：

• 让每一位患者获得正确的医疗结局；

• 吸引患者和人群参与；

• 患者参与医疗服务发展和供给的重要性；

• 患者的参与如何能改善医疗服务质量并提高医疗服务价值；

• 患者的参与如何能影响医疗资源分配和医疗资源匮乏之间的矛盾；

• 患者组织的重要性及双重角色。

■ 使每一位患者都能得到正确的医疗结局

改变有关"正确"患者结局的传统观点

数十年来，"正确"的定义建立于医学观念之上，直至 1972 年阿奇·科克伦出版其著作《效果和效力》（*Effectiveness and Efficiency*）[1]。科克伦的理论最初应用于医学实践中时被称为"临床流行病学"[2]。

随之，循证医学概念发展起来了[3]，它强调制定临床决策应基于当前最佳实证而非已经建立起来的医学观念。

循证医学（evidence-based medicine，EBM）要求把最佳研究证据、临床专家意见、患者个人价值观和具体情况整合在一起[3]。

个性化决策

对患者个体做出的"正确"诊疗是由临床医生和患者共同决定的。每百万人中，许多决策仅产生在每天就诊的 40 000 人中。这些决策或多或少在就诊时由临床医生和患者共同做出；但也有不少是由临床医生或患者本人在诊疗过程之外决定的，比如患者决定不服用为其开具的处方药物。每天的医疗决策总数很难估计，但是在每百万人口中可能会超过 200 000。这些决策对患者的医疗结果和费用都产生影响。

Although the development of evidence-based decision-making has increased the probability of a good outcome, evidence is only one factor in the clinical decision, as illustrated by the simple model of a treatment decision shown in Figure 1.11. From the patient's perspective, the need is for the right intervention, namely, an intervention for which there is a high probability of benefit and a low probability of harm, taking into account the unique clinical condition and values of the patient.

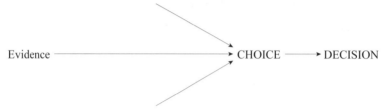

Figure 1.11   Relating the evidence to the needs and values of a particular patient

In the paradigm of evidence-based medicine, the use of best current evidence in decision-making is emphasised, but the clinician must also relate the evidence, which has often been produced during research studies on patients who are different from the type of patient seen in clinical practice, to the unique clinical needs of each patient. This task can be referred to as personalised medicine.

In addition, the development of our understanding of the human genome raises the possibility of using genetic tests to determine which particular treatment option would be best for a particular patient, an activity referred to as precision medicine or stratified medicine.

Preference-sensitive decisions

The third factor in any decision is the patient's values, that is, what value the patient places on the nature of the good and bad outcomes, and on the probabilities of each outcome occurring. In some clinical situations, the issues are clear, such as in the choice of treatment for fractured neck of femur. In others, such as in the treatment of prostate cancer, the different options for intervention have different consequences. To help patients make the decision that is best for them, it is essential they are given:

- *complete information about the probabilities of good and bad outcomes*
- *the opportunity to reflect on how these relate to their values*

尽管循证决策的发展提高了良好结局的概率，但正如图 1.11 治疗决策的简单模型所示，证据仅是临床决策中的因素之一。就特定临床状况和患者个体自身价值观而言，患者需要的是正确——即高获益、低损害——的医疗干预。

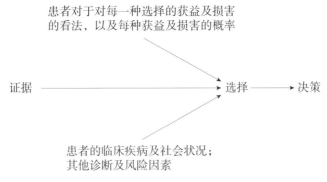

图 1.11　患者需求和价值观与医疗证据的关联

在循证医学的范式中强调将当前的最佳证据用于制订决策。但这些证据常常来源于那些与临床实际患者情况有差异的科学研究。临床医生必须将这些证据与每个患者实际医疗需求相结合，即所谓"个体化医疗"（personalized medicine）。

此外，随着我们对人类基因组研究的逐步深入，根据基因检测判定对特定患者效果最佳治疗方案的可能性也相应得到了提高，这被称为"精准医疗"（precision medicine）或"分层医疗"（stratified medicine）。

偏好敏感决策（preference-sensitive decisions）

在任何决策中的第三因素都指患者的价值观，即患者个人对结局好坏其发生概率的所持态度。在某些临床状况下，问题很容易解决，如股骨颈骨折的治疗选择；但在其他情况下，如治疗前列腺癌时，选择不同干预方案会带来不同的结局。因此，为帮助患者做出最佳决策，给予以下信息至关重要：

• 关于结局概率的详尽信息；
• 患者有机会考虑这些与个人价值观之间的关系。

The man considering different treatment options for prostate cancer needs support to reflect on whether it is more important for him to avoid incontinence or impotence. This principle holds true, even when the consequences of intervention are less dramatic. For example, in knee replacement, the patient needs to reflect on the degree of knee pain and stiffness they are currently experiencing and to consider the possibility that the operation may not be completely successful or could make the pain and stiffness worse. This type of decision has been called a preference-sensitive treatment decision.

> *Preference sensitive treatment decisions involve making value trade-offs between benefits and harms that should depend on informed patient choice. (4)*

In a report for the King's Fund in the UK, Mulley et al have called for an end to the 'silent mis-diagnosis' of patients (5), defined as the failure to diagnose the patient's preferences even though the clinician has diagnosed the disease accurately.

The need for patient decision aids

No fateful decision should be made in avoidable ignorance. (6) There is now a range of resources to improve decision-making, both for patients and clinicians, many of which were developed by the Foundation for Informed Medical Decision Making. The term given to the most structured of these decision-making tools is the patient decision aid.

To support patients and clinicians during shared decision-making, patient decision aids have been developed in recognition of the constraints that time places on face-to-face consultations. The consultation remains crucial because clinical judgement has an important part to play in identifying the patient's preferred style of decision-making; many patients still want their clinician to make the decision. The consultation, however, can be supplemented and complemented by decision aids.

There is now an extensive and strong evidence base about the problems patients face in making the choice that is right for them, and a growing evidence base about the steps that can be taken to improve a patient's decision-making (see Box 1.5). The steps to improve decision-making need to be managed as actively as the processes involved in the management of safety by the clinician responsible for a service.

男性患者在选择前列腺癌治疗方案时，需要得到支持，来考虑避免失禁或性功能障碍哪一个对于自身来说更为重要。即使干预结果并不严重，这一原则也需要得到贯彻。例如，膝关节置换术要考虑患者当前膝关节疼痛及僵硬的程度，还需考虑到该手术可能并非百分百会成功，甚至加剧疼痛僵硬的程度等。此类决策被称为偏好敏感决策。

偏好敏感决策包括利与弊之间的权衡，应该由患者在知情的情况下做出选择[4]。

在英国国王基金的一篇报告中，穆勒等人呼吁终结对患者"沉默的误诊"（silent mis-diagnosis）[5]，沉默的误诊是指：即使在疾病诊断准确的情况下，临床医生仍未能了解患者个人在治疗选择上的倾向。

患者决策辅助工具（patient decision aids）的必要性

应该避免在信息匮乏下做出重大决策[6]。当前有一系列资源都可以用来改善患者及临床医生的决策制定，其中很多都是由医疗知证决策基金会（Foundation of Informed Medicine Decision Making）提供的。在所有决策制定工具中，最成体系者被命名为"患者决策辅助工具"。

为了在医患共同决策过程中给予更好的支持，也由于人们意识到医患面对面诊疗时，时间有限，患者决策辅助工具得到了发展。即使有了患者决策辅助工具，医患之间的面对面诊疗仍至关重要；因为临床判断在确定患者偏好的决策方式中非常重要，多数患者仍希望由临床医生为自己做出决策，而决策辅助工具可面对面诊疗进行补充和完善。

当下已有了广泛有力的实证基础，让患者在面临问题时做出适合自己的选择；也有了越来越多的证据来改善患者决策的步骤（专栏 1.5）。改进决策的步骤需和安全管理相关过程一样，需要由负责医疗的医生进行积极管控。

Box 1.5 Steps that can be taken to improve decision-making (7)

- Presenting evidence about benefit or harm in relative terms rather than absolute terms results in the patients, and doctors, choosing different options. The use of absolute numbers, such as the number needed to treat (NNT), is more easily understood than presenting them in relative terms, such as relative risk. It is important to recognise that the research literature has a positive bias thereby giving the impression of greater benefit than is the case
- Offering all patients full information about the options because it is not possible to predict how much information a patient will want on the basis of their age or educational attainment. Giving full information in a way that suits the needs of individual patients will not increase the demand for resources. Indeed, evidence shows that it can decrease demand (5)
- Identifying patients' preferences for style of decision-making. Not all patients like the same style: some prefer to take the lead, some prefer the clinician to take the lead, and some prefer shared decision-making (8)
- Improving clinicians' skills in identifying the patient's preferred style of decision-making: many clinicians cannot discern which style of decision-making an individual patient prefers
- Using patient decision aids to help the patient weigh up the values they place on the benefits and the harms. Patient decision aids can also highlight the probabilities of each outcome and to overcome the constraints of time in face-to-face decision-making

It is clear, however, that many decisions are still made in 'avoidable ignorance'. Some of these fateful decisions concern elective surgery, others involve cancer treatment, and many are about end-of-life care. Indeed, the importance of distinguishing effectiveness and quality from outcome is particularly pertinent during end-of-life care. Many people receive effective, high-quality interventions when the outcome they most desire is a good death in their own home.

It is not possible to maximise value for a service and for a population without maximising the value for each individual patient.

■ Questions for reflection
- *In what way can patient decision aids help an individual patient make the decision that is right for them?*
- *What are the responsibilities for the clinician when ensuring that patients make the decision that is right for them?*

■ Engaging patients and populations

What's in a name: patients or principals?

Patients, customers, consumers, clients? We just call them punters.

专栏 1.5　可用于改善决策的步骤[7]

- 呈现结果损益证据时，相对术语优于绝对术语，方便患者和医生做出选择。而用绝对术语如"需治疗人数（number needed to treat，NNT）"比用相对专有术语如"相对风险（relative risk，RR）"，更易于被人们理解。要注意研究文献往往有正向偏倚，其显示的获益可能会优于实际情况。这一点十分重要。
- 因为无法通过患者年龄或受教育程度来预测其对信息的需求量，所以向所有患者提供可选方案的完整信息。提供能满足患者需求的完整信息并不会花费更多资源；事实上，有证据表明这反而可以降低需求[5]。
- 识别患者的决策偏好风格。患者的偏好风格各不相同：某些患者偏好由自己主导，某些偏好由临床医生主导，还有些则偏好共同决策[8]。
- 提高临床医生识别患者决策偏好风格的技巧：许多临床医生并不能辨别某患者在决策时的偏好风格。
- 用患者决策辅助工具来帮助患者权衡损益。患者决策辅助工具也会凸显每一种结果的概率，以克服医患面对面诊疗时决策时间不足的限制。

　　然而，许多决策仍然是在"可规避的无知"情况下做出的。某些重大决策涉及择期手术，有些则包括癌症治疗，还有很多涉及临终关怀。事实上，辨别结果的有效性和质量对临终关怀尤为重要。许多临终患者虽然接受了有效且高质量的干预，但他们最希望的往往是在自己家中平静离世。

　　脱离了患者个人价值的最大化，对一项服务和群体价值的最大化也就无从谈起了。

■ 思考题

- 患者决策辅助工具在哪些方面可帮助每个患者制定正确决策？
- 为确保患者决策正确，临床医生的职责是什么？

■ 让患者及人群也参与进来

我们该如何定位所服务的人？将其视为患者还是委托人？

　　　患者、顾客、消费者、客户？我们只把他们称之为赌博者。直

Let's face it, they are taking a chance every time they come into healthcare.

Doctor in Belfast

Patient: there is a move away from using this term; many professionals prefer to use 'citizen'. Alternatively, some professionals prefer to use terms such as 'people with diabetes' rather than 'diabetic patients' to ensure that a person is not characterised by their condition. In this section, the term 'patients' will be used as shorthand for people who have, or fear they have, a condition that could be helped by clinical intervention.

Principal: Economists often describe doctors as 'agents' because they act on behalf of the patient. The doctor (agent) is informed about a patient's health and their treatment options. The patient (principal) is relatively uninformed about these matters and therefore has to rely on the doctor to act in their (the patient's) best interests. A person will employ the services of an agent if they believe that their utility afterwards will be greater than without the help of the agent. (9)

From a legal perspective also, the patient is the principal, and the professional is the agent.

The new healthcare paradigm

Systems of care offer a new paradigm for healthcare in the 21st century. One of the changes brought in with this new paradigm is a shift from doctor- centred to patient-centred care. This shift is one of the most important aspects of the change in paradigm that is currently taking place (see Figure 1.12).

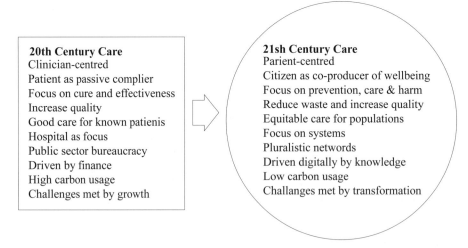

20th Century Care
Clinician-centred
Patient as passive complier
Focus on cure and effectiveness
Increase quality
Good care for known patienis
Hospital as focus
Public sector bureaucracy
Driven by finance
High carbon usage
Challenges met by growth

21sh Century Care
Parient-centred
Citizen as co-producer of wellbeing
Focus on prevention, care & harm
Reduce waste and increase quality
Equitable care for populations
Focus on systems
Pluralistic networds
Driven digitally by knowledge
Low carbon usage
Challanges met by transformation

Figure 1.12　The new healthcare paradigm for the 21st century

The implications of this shift are important for all clinicians irrespective of their different roles in relation to the population served, including:

面现实吧，他们每次接受医疗卫生保健服务时，都是经历一次博弈。

——来自贝尔法斯特的医生

患者：当前正倾向于避免使用这一词汇，许多专业人士倾向于称之为"公民"。或者，一些专业人士偏好使用"患糖尿病的人"而非"糖尿病患者"以避免用疾病来定义患者。在本章节，"患者"这个词被用于代指：患有或可能患有通过医学干预可缓解的疾病的人。

委托人：医生代表患者行事，因此经济学家经常将他们描述为"代理人"。医生（代理人）知情患者的健康状况及治疗选择方案，而患者（委托人）对此反而相对不知，因此不得不依靠医生为自己（患者）的最大利益行事。一个人雇佣代理是相信在该代理人的帮助下，自己能获得更大利益[9]。

从法律角度讲亦然，患者是委托方，而医疗专业人士则是代理人。

新型的医疗卫生保健范式

21 世纪医疗系统迎来了新型医疗卫生保健范式。这种新范式带来的改变之一，是医疗从原来的以医生为中心转变为以患者为中心。这可谓是正在运行的医疗范式最重要的转变之一（图 1.12）。

20世纪医疗
- 以医生为中心
- 患者为被动依从者
- 关注治疗和疗效
- 改善医疗服务质量
- 名人患病可得到更好的医疗
- 以医院为中心
- 官僚制度的公共部门
- 高碳使用
- 以金钱为驱动力
- 以扩张应对挑战

21世纪医疗
- 以患者为中心
- 公民为健康的共创者
- 关注预防、保健和伤害
- 减少浪费、改善质量
- 群体平等医疗
- 医疗体系为重点
- 多元化的网络
- 以知识驱动数字化
- 低碳使用
- 以转型应对挑战

图 1.12 21 世纪新型医疗卫生保健范式

不管临床医生在服务的人群中扮演着何种角色，这种以患者为中心的医疗模式的变化对所有临床医生来说都很重要。这种新模式需要：

• *caring for individual patients*

• *managing a service*

• *taking responsibility for the population of patients in need*

All clinicians need to adopt a new approach towards patients and understand the benefits that engaging patients will bring. Although one approach is to treat patients as equals in the healthcare transaction, this would not be sufficient because it is now accepted that patients have a major contribution to make to the development and delivery of health services.

The benefits of engaging patients

The main outcome of engaging patients is what is known as 'co-production'.

> *Co-production means delivering public services in an equal and reciprocal relationship between professionals, people using services, their families and their neighbours. Where activities are co-produced in this way, both services and neighbourhoods become far more effective agents of change. (10)*

Co-production can confer benefit in three domains of health service management:

• *engagement for performance improvement*

• *engagement in decision-making*

• *engagement to increase value*

Presenting these domains as a list does not show the potential for interaction and synergy, which is best conveyed diagrammatically (see Figure 1.13).

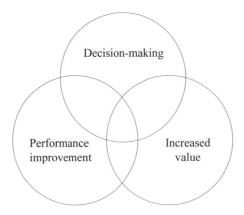

Figure 1.13   The three domains of health service management that benefit from patient engagement

- 为个体患者提供医疗卫生保健

- 管理每一项服务；

- 为有需要的患者群体负责。

所有临床医生都需要采用新方式对待患者，也需要理解患者的参与会给医疗带来益处。尽管其中的一种方式是在医疗过程中将患者放在与自己平等的位置上，但这还不够，因为现在普遍认为患者在医疗卫生保健的发展和实施的过程中都至关重要。

患者参与的益处

患者参与医疗的主要结果就是所谓的"医患共为"。

> "医患共为"指的是在医务工作者、医疗卫生保健接受者及其家人和邻里之间以平等互惠的关系提供医疗卫生保健。在那些以"医患共为"方式开展活动的地方，医疗卫生保健和相应的邻里都会成为更有效的变革推动者[10]。

医患共为能在医疗卫生保健管理方面带来以下三个好处：
- 参与绩效提升；
- 参与决策；
- 参与提高价值。

单纯的文字罗列不能体现三者之间交互协同的潜质，用图表的形式则可以很好地体现（图 1.13）。

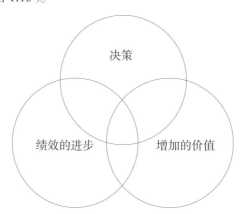

图 1.13　医疗服务管理因患者参与而受益的三个方面

Rules of engagement
- *The clinician responsible for the management of a clinical service has to relate to the patients currently in contact with that service*
- *The clinician responsible for population healthcare has to relate to all people in need, irrespective of whether they have been referred or are in contact with the service*

Engaging the patients seen by a clinical service

Throughout the book, we have emphasised the difference between managerial accountability for a service, that is, to the patients using the service, and accountability to a population, some of whom may be direct users of the service, while others are supported indirectly. This book focuses on the latter type of accountability for population medicine in which it is essential to use any opportunities to engage with patients. Engagement with people who are users of a specialist service reaches one part of the population. Although it is insufficient as a means of engaging the whole population in need, its potential should be realised by activities such as:

- *ensuring there are representatives of patients or carers on planning and development groups*
- *obtaining feedback from patients, for example, by using* www.iwantgreatcare. org or providing suggestion boxes
- *supporting the local branch of the relevant national charity*

Although these activities take place in many services and health centres at present, there is no engagement of those people in need who are not yet being cared for by the service. It is important to engage with the whole population in need.

Engaging with all the patients in the population

It is common to find that the patients being seen by a specialist service are not necessarily those who would benefit most from the service.

One response to this phenomenon is to increase the size of the specialist service; however, this may not be possible in an era of zero growth. Even if increased resources are available, simply providing more of the same would not maximise value. Instead, action needs to be taken:

- *to ensure that those people who will benefit most from specialist care are referred, for example, by providing training and guidelines to generalist clinicians such as domiciliary nurses, community pharmacists and general practitioners*
- *to increase the knowledge, skill and confidence of all clinicians treating the population so that generalists are able to care for a greater range of patients without referral to specialists. This requires the provision of*

参与规则

- 负责管理某项临床服务的临床医生只能让正在接受治疗者加入；
- 负责人群健康的临床医生，可以让所有有需求的人加入，无论是已被转诊者还是接受治疗者。

使接受临床服务的患者参与其中

在整本书中，我们一直在强调同一服务的两种管理职责之间的区别：一种是针对使用服务的患者；另一种是针对一个人群，该群体中一部分可能是直接使用者，而其他人则是间接的服务对象。本书关注的是后一种职责——群医学，有必要利用一切机会让患者参与其中。这已经在一部分专科医疗的使用者中实现。但这种方式还不能囊括整个有需求的群体，不过其潜力可通过以下活动表现出来：

- 确保在医疗规划和发展团队中有患者或照护者的代表；
- 获取患者的反馈，例如使用 www.iwantgreatcare.org 或提供意见箱；
- 支持国家相关慈善机构的地方分支机构。

虽然在许多医疗卫生服务中心中都在进行这些活动，但那些有需求却没得到医疗服务的人还没有参与其中。让整个有需要的群体都参与进来，这一点非常重要。

让人群中所有患者都参与其中

我们常常会发现，接受专科医疗服务的那些患者并不一定是从中受益最多的人。

一种应对这种现象的措施是提高专科医疗服务的规模，但是这种应对方式在医疗资源零增长的时代不太可行。即使医疗资源能有所增长，仅靠提供更多相同类型的医疗服务仍不能实现价值的最大化。因此我们应该采取以下措施：

- 让能从专科医疗服务中受益最多的人都被转诊到专科：比如为全科工作者——家庭护士、社区药剂师、全科医生等——提供培训和指南来实现此点；
- 所有对人群服务的医务人员都应丰富知识、增长技能和提高信心。这样就可使全科工作者能为更多患者提供医疗服务而无须把这些患者转

not only training but also the type of support that can be given easily by telephone and email

This approach will increase value from the resources available. It is also an expression of a new culture in which all healthcare professionals, generalists and specialists, work together to care for all the patients with a particular problem. The drawback is that this is a one-way process, from clinician to patient.

To complement the feedback that individual patients are able to give, either about the consultation they have just had or about the service as a whole, is the development of a working relationship between all clinicians and all patients and carers in the population, most easily through the relevant patients' organisations. Many patients' organisations already undertake a dual function (see Figure 1.14):

1.lobbying the body responsible for resource allocation for increased resources for their particular community of patients

2.helping the relevant service directly, not only by raising funds but also by providing peer-support for newly diagnosed patients and information for patients and carers

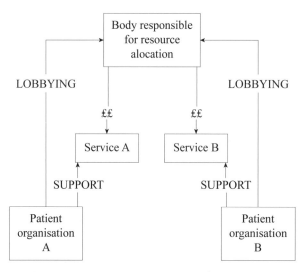

Figure 1.14   The dual role of patients' organisations

Supporting patients' organisations

Just as the individual patient is a partner in their care, the community of patients is a partner in the network that delivers services to them.

The clinician practising population medicine can engage with patients other than those in direct contact with the specialist service by supporting the relevant patient organisation (see Box 1.6).

诊至专科。这不仅需要为医务人员提供培训，还可采用更简易可行方法如通过电话和电子邮件等给予帮助。

此类举措可以提高现有可用资源的价值，也展现了一种新的医疗文化：即所有的医务人员、全科工作者和专科医生，一起为有特定医疗需求的患者提供服务。然而缺点是此过程是从医生到患者的单向过程。

补充患者的反馈意见——无论是对于刚结束的就诊还是对于整体服务评价——就是在人群中的所有临床医生、患者和护理人员建立工作关系。这最容易通过相关患者组织来完整。很多患者组织已经起到了类似的双重作用（图 1.14）：

- 游说负责医疗资源分配的机构，为特定的患者群体增加医疗资源；
- 为相关的服务提供直接的帮助，不仅是筹集资金，而且还为新确诊的患者提供同伴支持，并为患者和照护者提供相关信息。

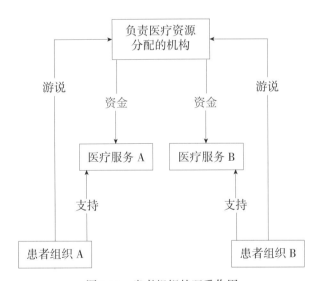

图 1.14 患者组织的双重作用

支持患者组织

正如患者个体是其医疗过程中的参与者，患者组织也是医疗服务实施网络中的一部分。

实践群医学的临床医生可以通过支持相关的患者组织、让所有患者参与进来，而非仅限于那些与专科医疗服务直接相关的患者（专栏 1.6）。

Box 1.6 Ways in which clinicians practising population
medicine can engage with patient organisations

- If a local branch of a patient organisation does not exist, ask the relevant national patient organisation to set one up
- Offer the local patient's organisation practical help, for example, by providing rooms for local meetings
- Offer to attend local meetings to ensure the organisation obtains best current knowledge about evidence from the published literature and about the services provided
- Participate in fundraising events for the organisation

Engaging the public

As resource allocation decisions are concerned with equity, or fairness, rather than efficiency (11), it is important to engage with the population that pays for healthcare when making them. There are two main types of resource allocation in which the public may become engaged during decision-making about service provision:

1. the allocation of resources within a service or programme, which is the responsibility of clinicians and managers working in each service who must engage with the patients who use that service and their representatives

2. the allocation of resources across services or programmes, which is the responsibility of those who pay for healthcare who must engage with the public as well as patients and their representatives

Although a patient organisation is focused on winning increased resources for the service or programme relevant to their members, it will have implications for other services. Similarly, there may be strong public reaction against proposed change to an individual service, such as the closure of a small but important paediatric service, even when the key healthcare professionals involved are in favour of the change.

If the public are not involved in the debate about resource allocation, the focus for argument may fall on one particular 'priority' after another, leading to demands that each should be funded. In the absence of a public appreciation that in allocating resources for one purpose, there is an opportunity cost, the results of which is that resources are denied to another group of patients.

By involving the public, and by definition their political representatives, in the debate and decision-making, those who pay for healthcare are able to shift the focus from being held to account for meeting every need to being held to account for the reasonableness of their decision-making. (12)

专栏 1.6　从事群医学的临床医生让患者组织参与进来的方法

- 如果当地没有患者组织的分支机构，则要求相关的国家患者组织在当地建立一个；
- 向当地患者组织提供实际帮助，如为举办会议提供场所；
- 主动参加当地的会议，以确保患者组织能在已出版的文献中获取有关证据的最新知识以及所提供医疗卫生保健的最新信息；
- 参加经费募集活动。

让公众参与其中

医疗资源配置决策关注的是平等或公平，而不是效率[11]。因此在制定这些决策时，让那些为医疗卫生保健付费的群体参与其中是非常重要的。在有公众参与的医疗服务决策过程中，主要有两种医疗资源分配类型：

- 对同一医疗卫生保健或项目的资源分配，是实施此项医疗卫生保健的医务人员和管理者的责任。他们必须让接受这项医疗卫生保健的患者及代表都参与其中；
- 对医疗卫生保健或项目之间进行资源分配，是医疗卫生保健付费者的责任。因此必须让公众、患者及其代表都参与其中。

尽管患者组织总是会努力为相关医疗服务项目或成员争取获得更多资源，但这也会对其他服务产生影响。与此类似，当提议更改个体的医疗服务时（如关闭某项小却重要的儿科服务），可能会遭到公众强烈反对，即使医疗卫生界重要人士对此投赞成票。

如果公众不能参与医疗资源分配的争论，则争论焦点就会落在一个又一个特定的优先项目上，从而出现认为每个优先项目都应该得到资金支持的呼声。如果公众不能取得为同一目标进行资源分配的共识，就会产生机会成本，其结果是拒绝把资源给另一个患者群体。

如果公众及其所指定的政治代表能参与讨论和决策，则为医疗卫生保健付费的人们就能将关注点从满足每项需求转到关注其决策的合理性上来[12]。

■ Questions for reflection

- *What are the disadvantages of engaging patients and their representatives in the management of services?*
- *What three points would you emphasise when making a presentation to a group of sceptical clinicians about increased engagement of patients?*
- *A patient group has nominated somebody to be their representative on a management team. They ask you for guidance about the duties of a 'patient representative' in this situation. Identify five points about the responsibilities this role would involve.*

─ References ─

Getting the right outcome for each individual patient

(1) Cochrane A. Effectiveness and Efficiency. United Kingdom: Taylor and Francis; 1972.

(2) Haynes RB, Sackett DL, Guyatt GH, Tugwell P. Clinical Epidemiology: How to Do Clinical Practice Research. 3rd Ed. Philadelphia: Lippincott Williams and Wilkins; 2004.

(3) Straus SE, Richardson WS, Glasziou P, Haynes RB. Evidence-Based Medicine. How to practice and teach EBM. 3rd Edition. Amsterdam: Elsevier Churchill Livingstone; 2005: 1.

(4) Christensen CM. The Innovator's Dilemma. New York: Harper Business Essentials; 2003.

(5) Mulley A, Trimble C, Elwyn G. Patients' Preferences Matter: Stop the Silent Misdiagnosis. London: King's Fund; 2012.

(6) Mulley A. Personal communication.

(7) O'Connor AM et al. Toward the 'Tipping Point': Decision aids and informed patient choice. Health Affairs. 2007; 26: 716–725.

■ 思考题

- 让患者及其代表参与医疗管理时，会有哪些弊端？

- 当你给那些对提高患者参与度持怀疑态度的医生作报告时，你会强调哪三点？

- 一个患者团体已经提名了某人担任其管理团队的代表，他们向你寻求关于这种情况下"患者代表"的职责指导，请给出这个角色责任的五个要点。

———————————————————————— 参考文献 —

(8) Gigerenzer G, Gray JAM. Better Doctors, Better Patients, Better Decisions. Massachusetts: MIT Press; 2010.

Engaging patients and populations

(9) Wonderling D, Gruen R, Black N. Introduction to Health Economics. Understanding Public Health. Maidenhead: Open University Press; 2005: 100.

(10) Boyle D, Harris M. Discussion Paper: The Challenge of Co- Production. How equal partnerships between professionals and the public are crucial to improving public services. London: NESTA; 2009: 11.

(11) Anand S. The Concern for Equity in Health. In: Anand, S., Peter, F. and Sen, A. (Eds). Public Health, Ethics and Equity. Oxford: Oxford University Press; 2004: 15.

(12) Daniels N, Sabin JE. Setting Limits Fairly, Learning to Share Resources for Health. Oxford: Oxford University Press; 2008: 44.

1.4 Towards value

In this section, we explore:

Maximising value and improving outcomes

- *the two different meanings of value – the moral meaning and the economic meaning*
- *the distinction between quality and value, and the relationship between those two concepts*
- *ways in which the allocation of resources, either between programmes or within a programme, can increase value*
- *how the management of innovation and redundancy is essential to maximise value*
- *the definition of inappropriate care and futile care*
- *how variations in practice may indicate the presence of inappropriate care*

Seven steps to increase value

- *the principal steps that can be taken to reduce the cost of population medicine*

Responsibility for reducing waste and increasing sustainability

- *muda and its relevance to population medicine*
- *a classification of different types of waste in healthcare*
- *a definition of sustainability*
- *the strategy that needs to be adopted to reduce the carbon footprint of clinical practice*

■ Maximising value and improving outcomes

The end of the quality era

For the last decade, the focus of healthcare managers and clinicians has been on quality improvement. As shown in Figure 1.15, focusing on quality alone improves, but does not maximise, value. Value is defined as doing the right things right to the right people.

There is now a shift in emphasis from quality to value. As with any paradigm shift, the new paradigm of increasing value encompasses the older paradigm of improving quality; however, it is necessary to clarify the meaning of the term 'value' in this context.

第 4 节　提升价值

在本节中，我们将探讨：

价值最大化与结局的改进

- 价值的两种不同含义——道德含义和经济含义；

- 质量和价值两者之间的区别与关系；

- 项目之间或内部资源分配的不同方式可以提升价值；

- 如何管理创新和冗余对价值最大化至关重要；

- 何谓不当和无效医疗照护；

- 实践中的差异如何能显示不当医疗卫生保健的存在。

提升价值的七个步骤

- 可降低群医学成本的关键步骤。

减少浪费和提高可持续性的职责

- 浪费及其与群医学的相关性；

- 医疗卫生保健中不同浪费形式的分类；

- 可持续性的定义；

- 需要采取策略以减少临床实践中的碳足迹①。

■ 价值最大化与结果改进

质量时代的终结

在过去十年中，医疗卫生管理人员和临床医生一直致力于改善质量。如图 1.15 所示，仅注重质量可以提高价值，但不能使价值最大化。价值被定义为"为正确的人做正确的事"。

现在的重点从质量转变为价值。与所有范式转变类似，提升价值的新范式是在旧范式的基础上的改进。然而有必要阐明本书中"价值"一词的含义。

---

① 是指一个人在各类日常活动过程中所引起的温室气体排放的集合。比如，日常用电、用油、用气，或是搭乘交通运输出行过程中所产生的碳耗量。碳耗量越多，排放量也就越大。

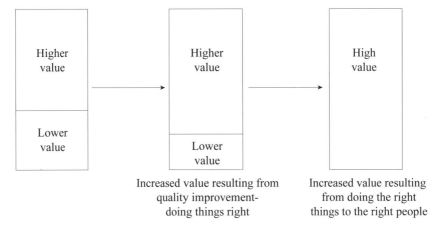

Increased value resulting from quality improvement-doing things right

Increased value resulting from doing the right things to the right people

Figure 1.15   Doing the right things right to the right people

The meanings of value

For an object, such as a book, it is possible to develop a definition stating what it is; however, for a concept, such as value, it is more productive to identify the various meanings of the term rather than to provide a definition.

There are many different meanings associated with the word 'value' when used in the context of healthcare.

The moral meaning: 'the status of a thing or the estimate in which it is held according to its real or supposed worth, usefulness, or importance' (a definition from late Middle English in the Shorter Oxford English Dictionary). This meaning of the word 'value', often used in the plural, is common in healthcare, for example, the hospital that states 'Our values are to promote patient choice', and 'We respect openness and honesty'. Another term to describe this meaning would be a 'principle'.

The economic meaning: one of the four variants of the term in the Shorter Oxford English Dictionary is 'that amount of some commodity, medium of exchange, etc. which is considered to be an equivalent for something else'.

In healthcare, value is measured by the relationship between outcome and cost, as expressed by the following formula:

$$Value = Outcomes/Costs$$

As any healthcare can do harm as well as good, the formula needs to be amended to reflect this:

$$Value = Good\ outcomes\text{-}bad\ outcomes/Costs$$

As good and bad outcomes are determined by the decisions and actions of professionals, the value of a service depends on:

• *whether decision-making is evidence-based*

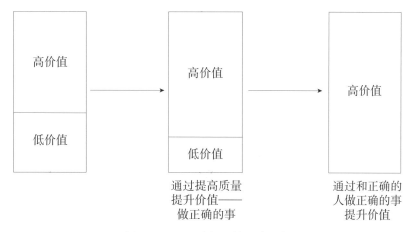

图 1.15　和正确的人做正确的事

价值的含义

对于书这样的物体而言，为其拟定一个定义说明其性质并非难事；然而，对于像价值这样的概念来说，剖析它的多重含义比单纯下定义更为复杂。

在医疗卫生保健领域中，"价值"一词有许多不同的含义。

道德含义："根据事情真实或应有的内涵、有用性或重要性而认为其应具备某个状态或估价。"（出自中世纪晚期《简明牛津英语词典》的英文定义）"价值观"这层含义多见于其英文名词的复数形式，在医疗卫生保健行业中很常见。比如，医院称"我们的价值观是优化患者的选择"，以及"我们尊崇开明守信的价值观"。而表达这个意思另外一个用词是"准则"。

经济含义：在《简明牛津英语词典》中，价值的四种含义之一是"某种商品的数量、交换的媒介（如货币、支票等）等，可被认为与其他某种东西等价"。

在医疗卫生保健领域中，价值由结局和成本之间的关系来衡量，如下公式所示：

$$价值 = 结局 / 成本$$

由于任何医疗卫生保健都可能有利有弊，因此需要对公式进行修订如下：

$$价值 = （好结局 - 坏结局） / 成本$$

专业人员的决策与行为决定了结局的好坏，而服务的价值取决于：

• 决策是否循证；

• *the safety of the service*

• *the quality of the service*

Although the paradigms of high-quality healthcare, evidence-based decision-making and patient safety remain important, the 21st century is the era of value in which the outcome is the dominant concern.

The meanings of outcome

Following the distinction of outcome from process by Avedis Donabedian, in the early literature on outcome, the most important step was to distinguish process measures from outcome measures. Process measures are easier to define and implement than outcome measures, but have less validity. For example, a process measure would be the degree to which a hospital achieved certain safety standards; the outcome measure would be a hospital's standardised mortality ratio (SMR).

During the last decade, the focus has shifted to the patient's perception of outcome. Initially, it was thought that patient experience measured service quality with greater validity than patient satisfaction, which is greatly influenced by a patient's expectations. It is now clear that the patient's opinion of the outcome of care must be measured and not simply the patient's experience of the interpersonal aspects of care. Thus, patient-reported outcome measures (PROMs) are seen as outcome measures at least as important as the clinician's perception of the success of an intervention.

The patient's perception of outcome has also become important in the context of an increasing emphasis on the 'harm of healthcare'. In the 20th century, the dominant preoccupation was the benefits of healthcare. In the 21st century, the dominant preoccupation will be the balance between benefit and harm, either from the perspective of the individual patient or from that of the population. In Matrix 1.2, the relationship between benefit and harm from an intervention for individual patients is shown.

		Benefits from intervention (good outcome)	
		Present	*Absent*
Harm from intervention (poor outcome)	*Absent*	Very good outcome	Disappointing for the patient: was the decision to intervene correct?
	Present	Perception of outcome dependent on the balance of good and harm and the patient's expectation when consenting (4)	Very bad outcome

Matrix 1.2　Relationship of benefit to harm for individual patients

- 服务的安全性；

- 服务的质量。

尽管高质量的医疗卫生保健、循证决策及患者的安全性这几方面依然很重要，但 21 世纪已进入以健康结局主导价值的时代。

结局的含义

在早期关于结局的文献中，阿维迪斯·多纳贝迪安指出结局和过程的区别，最重要的步骤是如何区分过程度量和结局度量。过程度量比结局度量更容易定义和实施，但效度较低。例如，过程度量可以是医院达到某些安全标准的程度；而结局度量可以是医院的标准化死亡率（SMR）。

在过去的十年里，患者对结局的看法越来越得到重视。最初，人们认为对于服务质量来说，患者体验的重要性高于患者满意度，因患者满意度受其期望的影响较大。现已明确的是，必须衡量患者对医疗卫生保健结局的看法和意见，且不只是患者接受了多少来自医务人员方面的关怀。因此，应把患者报告结局测量（patient-reported outcome measures，PROMs）与临床医生对干预成功的看法视为同等重要。

在日益强调医疗卫生保健危害的背景下，患者对结局的感受也变得十分重要。在 20 世纪，人们脑子里充满的都是医疗卫生保健带来的益处；而在 21 世纪，无论是患者个人还是公众，最主要的关注点都是利弊之间的平衡。矩阵 1.2 展示了患者个体干预中的利弊关系。

		干预产生疗效（良好结局）	
		有	无
干预造成损害 （不良结局）	无	良好结局	令患者失望：决定是否干预，是否正确
	有	对结局的看法取决于利弊的平衡和患者同意干预时的期望[4]	极差结局

矩阵 1.2　患者个体干预中的利弊关系

To ensure that a high proportion of patients have a good outcome, in addition to making sure that only interventions associated with strong evidence of doing more good than harm are delivered safely and at high quality, the clinician leading a service must take several different approaches:

- *to ensure that every patient facing a fateful decision makes it fully informed*
- *to ensure that the culture of the clinical service is one in which inappropriate or futile care is discouraged*

Lower-value healthcare

The fact that an intervention is effective, i.e. there is strong evidence that it does more good than harm, does not necessarily mean that it is of high value either to the population or to an individual. The value of an intervention depends on the context in which it is offered, which then determines whether its use is appropriate.

Assessments of the effectiveness of an intervention are objective, whereas assessments of the appropriateness of an intervention are subjective. Clinical judgement is used to place an intervention on the spectrum of appropriateness, from 'necessary' to 'futile' (see Figure 1.16).

NECESSARY   APPROPRIATE   INAPPROPRIATE   PUTILE

Figure 1.16   The spectrum of appropriateness

There are many definitions of all of the terms on the appropriateness spectrum: one of the definitions of a 'necessary' procedure is given by Kahan et al:

We define a procedure as necessary – or crucial – if all four of the following criteria are met:

- *The procedure must be appropriate*
- *It would be improper care not to recommend this service*
- *There is a reasonable chance that the procedure will benefit the patient. Procedures with a low likelihood of benefit but few risks are not considered necessary*
- *The benefit to the patient is not small. Procedures that provide only minor benefits are not necessary. (1)*

Kahan et al also offer definitions of 'appropriate' and 'inappropriate' in relation to a procedure:

... a procedure is termed appropriate if its benefits sufficiently outweigh its risks to make it worth performing, and it does at least as well as the next best available procedure. A procedure is termed inappropriate if the risks outweigh the benefits. (1)

为确保多数患者能获得良好结果，除了要将利大于弊的循证干预措施以保证安全、确保质量的方式提供给患者之外，临床医生还需采取一些不同的方法：

- 确保每个患者在面临重大决定时都能充分知情；
- 确保临床服务的文化是不鼓励采用不当或无效的医疗服务。

低价值的医疗卫生保健

某种有效的干预措施（例如，有强有力的证据表明其利大于弊）不一定意味着它对群体或个体都有很高价值。干预的价值取决于提供干预的环境，而环境又决定了干预是否适当。

对干预有效性的评估是客观的，而对干预适当性的评估是主观的。临床判断对干预措施适当性的范围从"必要"到"无效"（图 1.16）。

必要的	适当的	不当的	无效的

图 1.16　适当性的范围

适当性范围里的所有术语都有许多定义，卡汉等人给出了"必要"（necessary）程序的其中一个定义：

若能同时满足以下四个标准，我们则将此程序定义为必要或关键的：

- 程序必须适当；
- 不推荐这项医疗服务是不当的；
- 该程序有足够机会令患者受益。低风险低受益的程序则被认为是不必要的；
- 对患者的益处不应该小，只带来微小益处的程序被认为是不必要的[1]。

卡汉等人还给出程序"适当"和"不当"的定义：

　　……如果一项程序带来的益处远超过其风险，而且它至少应该与备选方案一样好，那么它是值得实施的，这个程序也是适当的。若其风险大于益处，则该程序是不适当的[1]。

Although it may be easy to agree upon the general definition of a term such as an 'appropriate' procedure, it is not as easy for a group of doctors to reach agreement when asked to identify whether an intervention is appropriate for a particular patient. Furthermore, it is not easy to reach an agreement on the definition of 'futility' when considered in relation to individual patients.

Clinicians may disagree about whether a procedure is appropriate or whether care is futile for a particular individual, but they tend not to be aware that the care offered by their service would be considered inappropriate by other doctors or people in other professional groups.

Two different types of data can highlight the possibility of inappropriate care:

- *time trends – as the rate of intervention increases, the probability of inappropriate care increases because treatment is offered to people who are less severely affected*
- *analysis of variation – widely differing rates of intervention in a population*

More is not necessarily better

Many elective operations are now performed much more frequently than they were in the past. For instance, the rate of cataract operations in England increased significantly from 1989 to 2004 (see Figure 1.17).

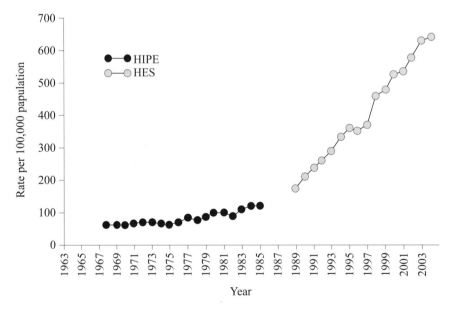

Figure 1.17   Rate of cataract operations per 100,000 population, 1989–2004

(reproduced from the British Journal of Ophthalmology, Tiarnan Keenan, Paul Rosen, David Yeates, Michael Goldacre, Volume 91, pages 901–904 © with permission from BMJ Publishing Group Ltd)

　　虽然在诸如"适当的"程序这类术语的一般定义上可能容易达成共识，但对于一些医生来说，一项干预对于特定患者来说是否合适就没那么容易达成一致意见了。此外，就患者个体而言，要就"无效"干预的定义达成一致并不容易。

　　临床医生可能就某特定患者的医疗程序是否适当或治疗是否无效存在分歧，但他们往往意识不到，其他医生或专业团体也会认为他们所提供的医疗服务不当。

　　两种不同类型的数据可以体现不当医疗服务的可能性：

- 时间趋势——干预率增加，不当医疗服务的可能性亦随之增加，因为可能会出现过度治疗；
- 差异分析：人群的干预率差异很大。

越多不一定越好

　　如今，许多非必需的手术比过去开展得更多了。例如从 1989 年到 2004 年，英国的白内障手术率就显著上升（图 1.17）。

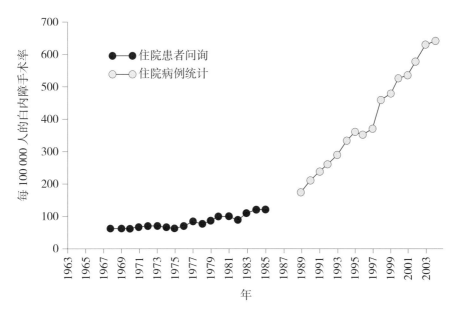

图 1.17　1989–2004 年每 100 000 人的白内障手术率

（引自 British Journal of Ophthalmology，Tiarnan Keenan，Paul Rosen，David Yeates，Michael Goldacre，91 卷，901–904 页，经 BMJ 许可）

Initially, an increase in the number of operations performed addresses what everyone would agree is unmet need, such that the increase in the volume of interventions provided is deemed necessary. With time, however, as the absolute number of operations and the rate of intervention increase, people whose need is less severe receive the intervention. In this instance it is debatable whether the care provided in this situation can be classified as 'necessary'.

Avedis Donabedian was the first to describe what happens when the volume of medical care provided to a population increases and the threshold for intervention changes. His description was originally published in Explorations In Quality Assessment & Monitoring (2), but latterly in Introduction to Quality Assurance in Healthcare (3). He pointed out that as the amount of resources invested increases:

- *the benefit that results from each unit of increase becomes smaller,* known as the Law of Diminishing Returns
- *the amount of harm done increases in direct proportion to the investment of resources, and follows the Law of Undiminished Harm (see Figure 1.18)*

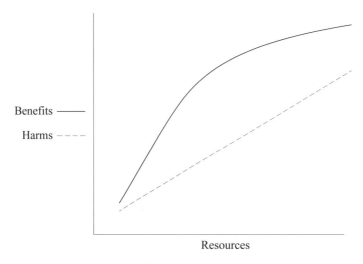

Figure 1.18   The Law of Undiminished Harm

Thus, there is a point when the investment of additional resources will lead to a reduction in net benefit or health gain calculated by subtracting the harm from the benefit. This is demonstrated in Figure 1.19. The turning point beyond which the investment of additional resources does not result in any increase in value Donabedian called the point of optimality.

Clinicians need to be aware of the point at which the balance between benefit and harm becomes unfavourable.

起初，手术量的增加解决了每个人未满足的需求，因此增加干预措施成为了必然之事。然而，随着时间推移，手术量和干预频率增加了，需求并不那么强烈的人也会得到干预。在这种情况下所提供的医疗服务是否"必要"则有待讨论。

阿维迪斯·多纳贝迪安首次说明了为人群提供的医疗服务增加并将更多人纳入干预范围会造成什么结果。他的研究最初发表在 *Explorations In Quality Assessment & Monitoring* 中[2]，后期又发表在 *Introduction to Quality Assurance in Healthcare* 上[3]。他指出，随着投入资源的增加：

• 每增加一个单位所产生的效益会变小，这就是收益递减规律；

• 所造成的损害程度与资源的投入成正比，并遵循损害递增规律（图 1.18）。

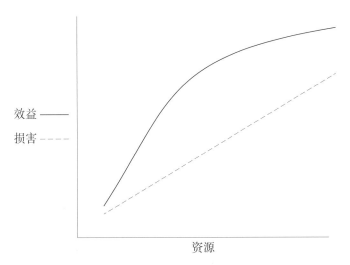

图 1.18　收益递减规律

因此，到了一定程度，额外的资源投入将导致净效益或健康收益的减少，其计算方法是从获益中减去损害。如图 1.19 所示。超过这个转折点，额外的资源投入不会带来任何的价值增加，多纳贝迪安称之为最优点。

临床医生需要意识到利弊平衡开始变得不利时的临界点。

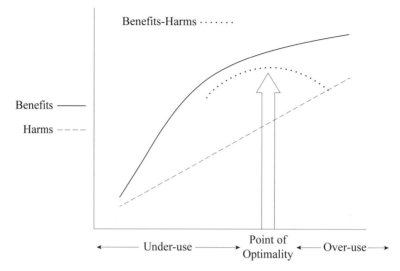

Figure 1.19 The relationship between resources, benefit and harm – under-use, optimality and over-use

Unknowing and unwarranted variation in practice

The groundbreaking research of Professor John Wennberg at Dartmouth Medical School demonstrated that there are large and unknown variations in clinical practice, such as in the rate of knee operations. Furthermore, much of this variation is not only unknown but also unwarranted, which he defined as:

Variation in the utilization of health care services that cannot be explained by variation in patient illness or patient preferences. (4)

It is important to appreciate that clinicians responsible for providing a greater level of intensity of care are convinced that the level of care is appropriate. No conscientious clinician provides inappropriate care consciously. Every clinician believes that what they deliver is appropriate but, because many clinicians and many local services work in isolation, there is little awareness of what others do. For this reason, the clinician intervening twice as often as the mean and the clinician intervening half as often as the mean believe they are intervening at the 'right' rate, as does the clinician who intervenes at the mean rate. None of them should necessarily be confident about the level of intervention, including the clinician intervening at the mean rate because that may encompass many inappropriate interventions.

The identification of inappropriate practice can be achieved in several ways:
- *by encouraging clinicians to visit other services or 'buddy' with another service so that exchanges can be arranged – working in another service can be illuminating*

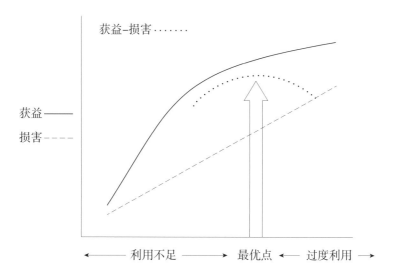

图 1.19 资源、获益和损害之间的关系——利用不足、优化和过度利用

临床实践中的未知和不合理的差异

达特茅斯医学院约翰·温伯格教授的一项开创性研究表明，在临床实践中存在着巨大且未知的差异，例如膝关节手术率。此外，此类差异大多数不仅是未知的，而且是不合理的，他将其定义为：

> 使用医疗卫生保健过程中不能用患者病情或患者偏好来解释的
> 差异[4]。

负责提供更高强度医疗服务的临床医生确信他们所提供的强度是合适的，意识到这点非常重要。尽责的临床医生绝不会故意提供不当的医疗服务。尽管每个临床医生都认为提供的医疗服务是适当的，但由于许多临床医生和地方服务机构是相互独立运作的，所以他们并不了解其他人的做法。因此，采取的干预强度是均值的两倍或一半的临床医生们都会认为自己是以"正确"的强度进行了干预。医生有时应该怀疑自己是否采用了自认为合理的干预强度（尽管仅采用了平均强度），因为这可能会造成许多不当干预。

不当干预的鉴别可以通过以下几种途径实现：

- 鼓励临床医生走访其他机构或兄弟单位，以便开展交流——了解不同机构可能会带来启发；

• *through peer-review of cases and case-notes*
• *by identifying and investigating variation in activity – the possibility that there is over-use or under-use of a service is raised if rates of activity are higher or lower than in comparable services caring for similar populations*

As discussed, the appropriateness of an intervention is distinct from its effectiveness. Appropriateness is determined by the values of the patient. Therefore, it is essential that the patient's values are incorporated into any clinical decision about whether or how to intervene. This can be done by promoting shared decision-making through the use of patient decision aids.

Variations analysis and shared decision-making are both ways in which the 'right' outcomes can be achieved for populations and individual patients, respectively. Furthermore, these methods are inter-related. When rates of intervention are high, the balance of benefit to harm may be beyond the point of optimality from a population perspective. From the perspective of an individual patient, the types of outcome that have to be considered are also different because, as Wennberg highlighted, when there are more resources:

• *less severely affected people are being offered interventions*
• *for each person, the magnitude of benefit that can be expected is reduced because their problem is less severe to start with, however, the likelihood and magnitude of harm experienced is the same as for more severely affected people*

Wennberg states that if an operation is performed on a patient who does not understand the risks they face, and who would not have accepted the offer of the operation if they had been so informed, the service has operated on 'the wrong patient'.

■ Seven steps to increase value

Although steps to improve quality and safety as core functions of service management lead to better outcomes, there are further steps that a clinician responsible for delivering healthcare to a population can take to increase value (see Box 1.7).

Box 1.7 Seven steps to increase value in healthcare

1. Negotiating well with payers and commissioners

2. Allocating resources to different patient groups to achieve optimality

3. Within each group of patients with the same condition, allocating resources to achieve the optimal balance of prevention, diagnosis, treatment and care

4. Ensuring the right patients are seen by the service

5. Encouraging innovation and disinvestment to increase value

6. Getting the right outcome for the right patient

7. Reducing waste

- 开展病例和病历记录的同行评议；

- 辨别和调查活动中的差异——如果某项服务的活动率高于或低于针对类似人群的同类服务，则会增加该项服务过度利用或利用不足的可能性。

如前所述，干预的适当性不同于其有效性。适当性由患者的价值观决定。因此，将患者的价值观融入临床决策（是否或如何干预）中是至关重要的。可以通过应用患者辅助决策工具来促进共同决策。

差异分析和共同决策两种方法都可以使得患者群体和个体获得"正确"结果。此外，这些方法是相互关联的。当干预率很高时，从群体的角度来看，利弊平衡可能会超过最优点；从个体的角度来看，需要考虑的结局也是有所不同的，因为正如温伯格强调的，当资源更多时：

- 病情较轻者也会得到干预。

- 对每个人而言，由于其问题从一开始就不太严重，所以结局很难如预期一样好，但其受到伤害的可能性和程度与病情更重的人却相差无几。

温伯格指出，如果对不了解手术风险的患者进行了手术，而当其充分知情后可能选择不接受手术，那么这个手术就"找错了患者"。

■ 提升价值的七个步骤

虽然改善服务管理的核心功能即质量和安全性会带来更好的结果，但负责人群健康的临床医生还可以采取进一步的措施来提升价值（专栏 1.7）。

专栏 1.7　提升医疗卫生保健价值的七个步骤

1. 与费用支付者和委托人进行良好的谈判。

2. 将资源分配给不同的患者群体，以达到最优效果。

3. 在每一组病情相同的患者中，分配资源以达到预防、诊断、治疗和保健的最佳平衡。

4. 确保那些真正有需求的患者得到服务。

5. 鼓励创新并减少投入以提升价值。

6. 让正确的患者能够得到正确的健康结局。

7. 减少浪费。

Step 1: Negotiating well with payers and commissioners

Those who pay for or commission healthcare are responsible for allocating resources to different programme budgets. The allocation of resources in NHS England across 23 programme budget categories is shown in Table 1.2. (5)

One of the key responsibilities for the clinician managing a service is to try to gain additional resources from the organisation that allocates money to all programmes of care. In an era of constraint, this responsibility may become one of trying to prevent the service from suffering cuts.

In times of growth, clinicians managing services have become accustomed to bid for resources to add to the programme budget for their service, relying on the institution allocating resources among programmes to fund in their favour based on the case of need submitted. The case of need, or business case, has traditionally been based on evidence of effectiveness and cost-effectiveness.

Table 1.2 Programme budgeting estimated England-level gross expenditure for programmes in 2010/11

Programme budgeting category code	Programme budgeting category	Gross expenditure 2010/11 (£ billion)
1	Infectious Diseases	1.80
2	Cancers & Tumours	5.81
3	Disorders of the Blood	1.36
4	Endocrine, Nutritional and Metabolic Problems	3.00
5	Mental Health Disorders	11.91
6	Problems of Learning Disability	2.90
7	Neurological	4.30
8	Problems of Vision	2.14
9	Problems of Hearing	0.45
10	Problems of Circulation	7.72
11	Problems of the Respiratory System	4.43
12	Dental Problems	3.31
13	Problems of the Gastro- Intestinal System	4.43
14	Problems of the Skin	2.13
15	Problems of the Musculo- Skeletal System	5.06

第一步：与支付者和委托人进行良好的谈判

那些支付或委托医疗卫生保健服务的人负责将资源分配给不同项目预算。英国国家医疗服务体系在 23 类项目预算上的资源分配情况见表 1.2 [5]。

临床医生在服务管理中的关键职责之一是设法从那些为所有医疗服务项目拨款的机构中获得额外资源。在一个资源稀缺的时代，这种职责可能会是尽量不让卫生保健服务被砍掉。

在经济增长时期，管理服务的临床医生已经习惯于竞标资源以增加其服务的方案预算。机构会根据提交的需求为他们偏爱的项目分配资源。需求案例或项目企划通常是根据有效性和成本效益的证据来决定的。

表 1.2 2010/11 年度英国医疗服务项目的预算

项目预算类别编号	项目预算类别	2010/11 年度总支出（亿英镑）
1	感染性疾病	18.0
2	癌症和肿瘤	58.1
3	血液疾病	13.6
4	内分泌、营养和代谢疾病	30.0
5	精神健康障碍	119.1
6	学习障碍	29.0
7	神经系统疾病	43.0
8	视力障碍	21.4
9	听力障碍	4.5
10	循环系统疾病	77.2
11	呼吸系统疾病	44.3
12	口腔疾病	33.1
13	消化道疾病	44.3
14	皮肤病	21.3
15	肌肉－骨骼系统疾病	50.6

continued

Programme budgeting category code	Programme budgeting category	Gross expenditure 2010/11 (£ billion)
16	Problems due to Trauma and Injuries	3.75
17	Problems of the Genito- Urinary System	4.78
18	Maternity and Reproductive Health	3.44
19	Conditions of Neonates	1.05
20	Adverse Effects and Poisoning	0.96
21	Healthy Individuals	2.15
22	Social Care Needs	4.18
23	Other Areas of Spend/Conditions	25.95
Total		107.00

Let us take the situation among three programme budgets – respiratory disease, gastro-intestinal disease and cancer – as an example. The respiratory services programme has bid for additional resources. If successful, the respiratory services programme would receive an increased amount of resources and thereby a greater proportion of the budget, whereas the services for people with gastro-intestinal disease and cancer would retain the same absolute amount of resources but receive a smaller proportion of the budget. When making decisions about resource allocation among different programmes of care, decision-makers have to take as a starting position the inherited levels of resource allocation (see Figure 1.20).

In times of fiscal constraint when there is no growth in resources, those paying for healthcare and commissioners have to switch resources from one programme budget to another, using a process called marginal analysis.

The aim is to achieve Pareto optimality, that is, the point at which allocative efficiency is at its maximum when the distribution of resources is such that shifting a dollar from one budget to any other would produce no more value. Needless to say, this state of Pareto optimality has never been reached in any health service. The allocation of resources across programme budget categories in NHS England (see Table 1.2) may not necessarily result from a process of logical analysis, but instead be the end result of decades of ad-hoc decision-making.

续表

项目预算类别编号	项目预算类别	2010/11 年度总支出（亿英镑）
16	外伤和创伤疾病	37.5
17	生殖泌尿系统疾病	47.8
18	产妇和生殖健康	34.4
19	新生儿健康	10.5
20	不良反应和中毒	9.6
21	有关个体健康	21.5
22	社会关怀需求	41.8
23	其他领域的支出 / 问题	259.5
合计		1070.0

以呼吸系统疾病、消化道疾病和癌症 3 个项目预算为例。针对呼吸系统的医疗服务项目已竞标获得了额外资源。顺利的话，呼吸系统医疗服务项目将获得更多的资源，从而在财政预算中占更大的比例；而为胃肠道疾病和癌症患者提供的医疗服务的绝对数量可能不会变化，但在预算中所占的比例可能会减少。当决策者在不同的医疗服务项目之间分配资源时，应该参照最开始的资源配置水平（图 1.20）。

在财政紧张时资源总量难以增长，那些用于支付医疗卫生保健和专员的费用就需要从一个项目转移到另一个项目，所依据的是边际分析方法。

该方法的目标是实现"帕累托最优"。所谓的帕累托最优可以理解为：当从一项预算中转移一美元到其他任何预算中将不会产生更多价值时，配置效率已达到最大。毋庸赘言，任何医疗服务中都未曾实现过帕累托最优。英国国家医疗服务体系（NHS）跨项目预算类别的资源分配（表 1.2）不一定是逻辑分析过程的结果，而是几十年临时决策的最终结果。

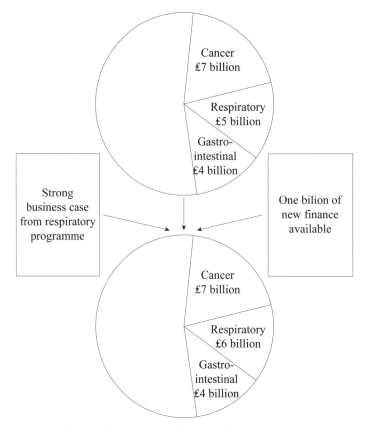

Figure 1.20   Winning resources for the respiratory programme budget
when resources are increasing

In future, the clinician responsible for delivering a service to one subgroup of the population will have to prepare a bid or business case in which it is argued that:

- *there is no waste or lower-value activity in their budget*
- *if resources were switched from another programme budget, the population as a whole would receive better value (Figure 1.21)*

Before embarking on marginal analysis, however, those who pay for healthcare and commissioners will expect clinicians to examine their own budgets, and to receive assurance that:

- *the entire programme budget is allocated optimally to the different conditions within that programme*
- *the service achieves high value from the resource allocation*

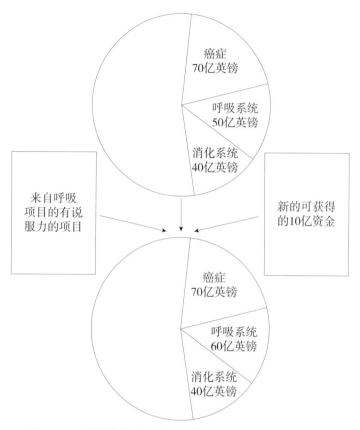

图 1.20　当赢得资源时，呼吸系统服务项目获得了更多预算

　　未来，负责向人群中的亚人群提供服务的临床医生必须准备一份投标书或商业企划，其中需要说明以下几点：

- 他们的预算中没有浪费或低价值的活动；
- 从另一个项目预算中调拨资源，他所负责的整个人群将获得更好的价值（图 1.21）。

　　然而，在进行边际分析之前，那些医疗卫生费用的支付者和委托人期望临床医生检查他们自己的预算，并保证以下内容：

- 整个项目预算在该项目内的不同条件下得到最优分配；
- 通过资源分配实现服务的高价值。

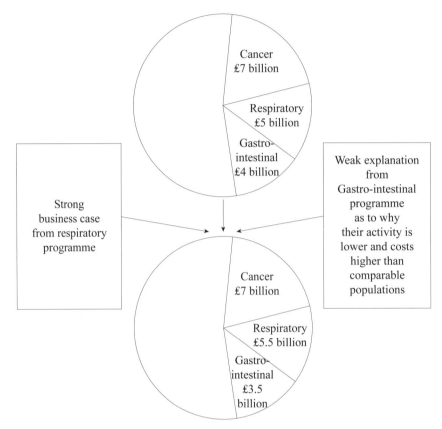

Figure 1.21　Winning resources for the respiratory programme budget when there is no growth in resources

Step 2: Allocating resources to different patient groups optimally

Unless general practitioners have a special interest in a particular condition or aspect of medicine, as generalists they need to distribute their resources among all their patients as best they can, given that they deal with all types of health problem. Specialists, however, are frequently faced with more explicit decisions about the allocation of resources among a small number of patient groups or subspecialties, although specialists also have to take account of patients with rare diseases.

When there are increases in health service investment, the clinician who is a manager bids for more resources to increase the amount invested in the condition for which increased need has been identified, such as in a sleep apnoea service where need has increased due to improved diagnosis and the development of new technology. When there is no increase in health-service investment, the most likely source of additional finance for sleep apnoea will be from within the respiratory diseases programme budget (see Figure 1.22), which in England is about £100 million per million population.

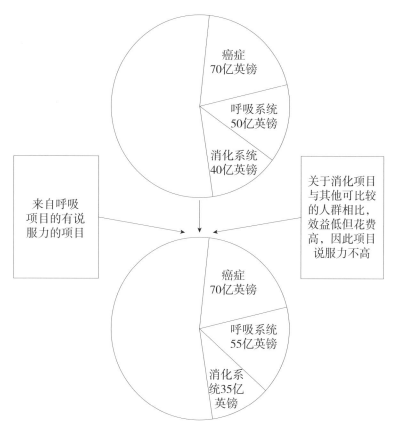

图 1.21　在资源没有增加的情况下，为呼吸系统的服务项目赢得了更多预算

第二步：将资源分配给不同的患者群体，以达到最优效果

除非全科医生对某一疾病或医学某一方面有特殊兴趣，否则，鉴于他们要处理各种类型的健康问题，他们需要尽可能地把资源分配给所有患者。与全科医生不同的是，专科医生最常面临的问题是如何在不多的几组患者之间或各组亚专科之间分配资源有时还需要考虑罕见病患者群体。

当医疗卫生保健服务投资增加时，作为管理者的临床医生会为已确定需要增加需求的服务内容竞标，以争取更多的资源。例如，诊断技术的改进和新技术的发展导致睡眠呼吸暂停综合征的相关服务需求增加时，医生就可以寻求增加这方面的资源。当医疗卫生保健投资没有增加时，睡眠呼吸暂停综合征的额外资金将最可能来自呼吸系统疾病的项目预算（图 1.22），在英格兰，这一预算约为每百万人口 1 亿英镑。

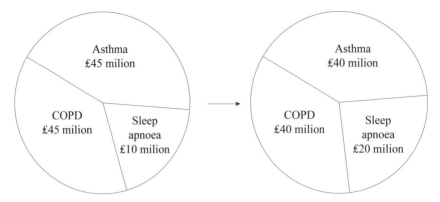

Figure 1.22   Finding resources for sleep apnoea from within the Respiratory
Programme Budget (figures are approximations)

It is rare that the decision-maker is able to make a decision completely rationally. They must use what Herbert Simon called 'bounded rationality', a principle that the main proponents of systems thinking have adapted and promoted.

> *The capacity of the human mind for formulating and solving complex problems is very small compared with the size of the problem whose solution is required for objectively rational behaviour in the real world of even for a reasonable approximation to such objective rationality. (6)*

In making decisions about the care for a population, such as the population of Christchurch, New Zealand, or a subgroup of the population with common needs such as people with respiratory disease, three factors have to be taken into consideration (see Figure 1.23):
- *evidence of good and bad effects of all the interventions*
- *the value the population places on the benefits and harms of each care option*
- *the other needs of the population*

The value the population places on benefits and
harms of each of the care options

Evidence
of good and
bad effects ⟶ → CHOICE ⟶ DECISION
of all the
interventions

The other current needs
of the population

Figure 1.23   Relating the evidence to the needs and values of the population

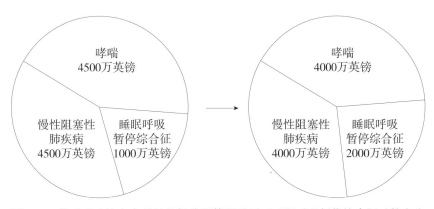

图 1.22   将呼吸系统疾病项目的部分预算调整用于睡眠呼吸暂停综合征（数字为近似值）

决策者很少能够完全理性地做出决定。他们必须使用赫伯特·西蒙所称的"有限理性"（bounded rationality），这是系统思维倡导者已经习惯遵循并提倡的原则。

> 与所需要解决的问题规模相比，人类头脑发现和解决复杂问题的能力非常小，这些问题的解决方案需要现实世界中客观理性的行为，或者是近似这种客观理性的行为[6]。

在对某人群（如新西兰的克赖斯特彻奇人）或有共同需求的某个亚人群（如呼吸系统疾病患者）进行医疗服务决策时，必须考虑三个因素（图 1.23）：
- 所有干预措施所产生影响（正面的、负面的）的证据；
- 人群对每种医疗服务选择的利弊持有的价值观念；
- 人群的其他需要。

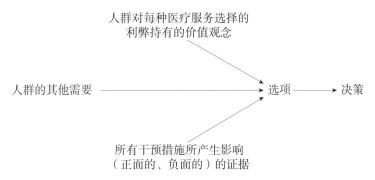

图 1.23   将证据和人群的需要及价值取向联系起来

As the evidence is rarely 100% conclusive and it is impossible to model precisely the impact of the resources used on the whole population, the decision-maker will have to make a value judgement. Judgement is a subtle concept that has more than one meaning. Furthermore, value judgements often have important ethical elements. Thus, judgement is exercised not only in weighing the different options but also in understanding, calculating and managing the ethical elements of the decision. This complexity has been described by Herbert Simon.

> *It is here that judgement enters. In making administrative decisions it is continually necessary to choose factual premises whose truth or falsehood is not definitely known and cannot be determined with certainty with the information and time available for reaching that decision...*
>
> *In ordinary speech there is often confusion between the element of judgement in decision and the ethical element. This confusion is enhanced by the fact that the further the means-end chain is followed, i.e. the greater the ethical argument, the more doubtful are the steps in the chain, and the greater is the element of judgement involved in determining what means will contribute to what ends. (7)*

This exercise of judgement can bring the clinician responsible for the budget into conflict with colleagues, particularly if those colleagues do not feel any responsibility towards the stewardship of resources. In this situation, it can be helpful to provide colleagues with examples of types of activity that can be classified as being of lower value to populations and patients (see Box 1.8).

Box 1.8 Interventions or services of lower value

- There is clear evidence of ineffectiveness or evidence that the interventions do more harm than good
- There is no or weak evidence of effectiveness but the intervention/service is not being delivered in a context that would enable the collection of evidence to judge effectiveness, e.g. not being delivered as part of an ethically approved, well-designed research project – these interventions are often referred to as 'innovations' or 'developments'
- There is evidence of effectiveness, but the intervention/service is being offered to patients whose characteristics are different from those of the patients in the original research studies that produced the evidence of effectiveness
- The interventions consume resources that would produce more value, i.e. a better balance of benefit to harm, if invested in another intervention/service for the same group of patients

由于证据几乎不能百分百确定，加上也不可能精确地估计出所使用资源对整个人群的影响，因此决策者必须对价值做出判断。判断是一个微妙的概念，有不止一种含义。此外，价值判断往往具有重要的伦理因素。因此，判断不仅要权衡不同选择，而且需要考虑对决策的理解、计算、管理以及伦理因素。赫伯特·西蒙曾描述过这种复杂性。

这就需要判断了：在行政决策中，需要不断对事实前提进行选择；但我们无法判断这些事实前提的真伪，也无法根据现有信息判断其确切性，留给我们决策的时间也很紧迫……

在日常对话中，常常会混淆决策判断因素和伦理因素。这种混淆因为以下事实而加剧：如果遵循方法 – 目的链，也就是说，道德争论越激烈，在通过方法实现目的的推导链条上的因素就越可疑，因此，在决定采用何种手段以利于实现何种目的时，所需考虑的判断因素也就越多[7]。

这种判断会使负责预算的临床医生与同事间发生冲突，特别是当这些同事对资源管理不承担任何责任时。在这种情况下，向同事举例说明那些对人群和患者价值较低的活动类型可能会有助于他们对情况的理解（专栏 1.8 ）。

专栏 1.8　价值较低的干预或服务

- 有明显的证据表明这些干预措施并无效果或弊大于利。
- 没有有效证据或仅有弱的有效证据，造成此情况的原因是此干预是在缺少可以判断其有效性的情景下进行的，或者说实施此干预的研究项目不符合伦理要求，在设计上有缺陷。这种干预或服务项目往往被称为有创新性或发展性。
- 证据表明其有效，但被提供干预 / 服务的患者与原始研究中证明有效的患者对象人群特征不同。
- 如果对同一组患者施以另一种干预照护，其消耗的资源会产生更多的价值，且能在利弊间得到更好的平衡。

Step 3: Achieving optimal balance between prevention, diagnosis, treatment and care for a single group of patients

Value-based decisions also have to be made when considering a single group of patients – people with chronic obstructive pulmonary disease (COPD), for example. Decision-making about care for a group of patients can include a value judgement because:

- *the options are rarely directly comparable*
- *each option may be championed by an enthusiast for their particular intervention, ready to argue why they need more resources or why they should be spared a cut*

This process of achieving an optimal balance in resource allocation for a single group of patients is referred to as 'within-system marginal analysis'. In this type of marginal analysis, the options must be considered within the limits of the finite resources available for that particular health problem. For instance, the clinician in charge of respiratory services for a population who has already allocated all the resources optimally to the three principal conditions – asthma, sleep apnoea and COPD – may have to use judgement to decide on the balance of resources between treatment and rehabilitation.

Consider the options facing the clinician responsible for a comprehensive COPD service. They can allocate resources to five different types of intervention – prevention, diagnosis, treatment, rehabilitation and end-of-life or palliative care (see Figure 1.24). The smallest proportion of funding is for prevention ('Smoking cessation'), but is that the lowest source of value? The decision to switch resources from treatment to prevention, or vice versa, is a value judgement encompassing ethical elements, as is the decision to switch resources from asthma to COPD or from respiratory disease to cancer.

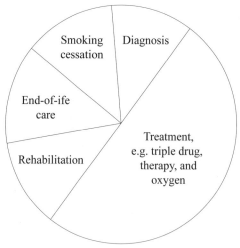

Figure 1.24 Components of the system budget for COPD

第三步：在同一病种患者之间实现预防、诊断、治疗和照护最佳平衡

当考虑同一病种患者群体时（例如慢性阻塞性肺疾病患者），也需要基于价值的决策。对同一病种患者的医疗卫生保健服务决策也包括价值判断，其原因是：

- 这些选项几乎不具有直接的可比性；
- 每一种选择都可能被特定干预措施的狂热者所倡导，他们随时准备为争取更多资源或避免被削减的缘由而争论不休。

为某同一病种患者取得资源分配的最佳平衡的过程可被称为"系统内边际分析"。在这种边际分析中，必须在针对特定健康问题的有限资源范围内考虑各种选择。例如，对于已经将所有资源以最优方式分配给三种主要疾病：哮喘、睡眠呼吸暂停综合征和慢性阻塞性肺疾病的人群时，负责呼吸系统医疗卫生保健的临床医生可能不得不判断治疗和康复之间的资源平衡。

当临床医生提供慢性阻塞性肺疾病综合医疗卫生保健时，可能会遇到不同的选择，他们可以将资源分配到五种不同类型的干预——预防、诊断、治疗、康复和临终或姑息治疗（图 1.24）。资金比例最小的是用于预防（"戒烟"），但这是价值最低的部分吗？决定将资源从治疗转投向预防，就像决定将资源从哮喘转向慢性阻塞性肺疾病或从呼吸道疾病转投向癌症（反之亦然），是一个包含各种伦理因素在内的价值判断。

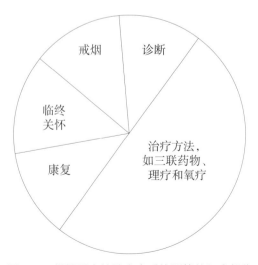

图 1.24　慢性阻塞性肺疾病系统预算的组成部分

To support clinicians in the allocation of resources within a service, tools have been developed by a team at the London School of Economics (LSE) that can enable the value of different choices to be estimated and displayed in order to stimulate discussion and debate. (8)

Step 4: Ensuring the right patients are seen

One of the most important actions in population medicine is to ensure that a specialist service sees the right patients, and that the patients being supported by generalists receive the right care. This requires the clinician practising population medicine to be concerned about all the people in the population who have a particular condition, and to support all the clinicians working with that population irrespective of whether those clinicians are generalists or specialists.

Taking a population approach to health services is likely to reduce inequity because there is usually a higher proportion of people from disadvantaged and deprived communities in the subgroup of the population who are either not seen by the specialist service or who do not receive a particular intervention.

Step 5: Encouraging innovation and disinvestment to maximise value

Another way of classifying the value judgements that a clinician responsible for delivering services to a population has to make is to consider them as investment or disinvestment decisions. Decisions about investment or disinvestment are generated by the desire to fund an innovation created by either another organisation, such as a new drug or a new piece of equipment, or someone who works in or uses the service (see Figure 1.25).

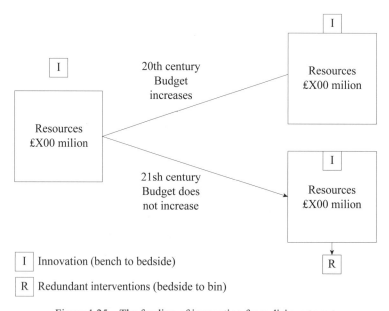

Figure 1.25　The funding of innovation from disinvestment

为了支持临床医生在服务中对资源的分配，伦敦政治经济学院（LSE）的团队开发了一些工具，可以估算和展示不同选择的价值，从而促进讨论和辩论[8]。

第四步：确保那些正确的患者得到服务

群医学最重要的行动之一是确保专科医生能够看到正确的患者，并确保接受全科服务的患者能得到正确的医疗服务。这要求从事群医学的临床医生关注人群中患有特定疾病的所有患者并支持治疗这些患者的全部临床医生，无论他们是全科医生还是专科医生。

用针对人群开展医疗卫生保健服务的方法和手段可以减少不平等。因为在弱势人群和贫困社区一类的亚人群中，有较高比例的居民既没有得到专科医疗服务也没有得到特殊干预。

第五步：鼓励创新并减少投入以实现价值最大化

另一种价值判断的分类方法是，当负责向人群提供服务的临床医生作决策时，必须将价值判断视为投资或撤资的决定。有关投资或撤资的决定是为了投资另一项目（比如新药或新设备）或另一人（使用该服务或为其工作）的创新项目（图 1.25）。

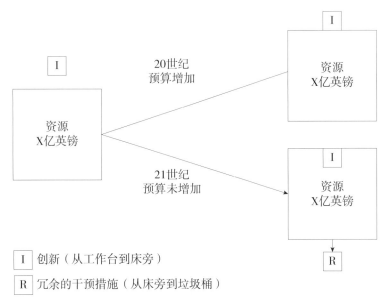

I　创新（从工作台到床旁）

R　冗余的干预措施（从床旁到垃圾桶）

图 1.25　减少投资为创新提供资金

Encouraging higher-value and discouraging lower-value innovation

Innovation is usually associated with starting new services or procedures; however, two other activities are of greater importance if innovation is to be managed well:

- *stopping starting – that is, stopping the drift into practice of lower-value interventions*
- *starting stopping – that is, stopping lower-value activities so that resources may be released for re-use, referred to as disinvestment*

Those who manage clinical services have to be alert to the arrival of new technology that does not increase value or, if it does, is introduced before other interventions deemed to be of lower value have been stopped or scaled down. Controlling procurement and the order book allows new technology to be appraised. It is possible, however, for new technology to bypass appraisal processes in various ways:

- *through being lent by the developer*
- *by masquerading as research*
- *by being given by the manufacturer without an initial charge in an attempt to change clinical practice*
- *by being bought by a charity in an attempt to change clinical practice*

Those who manage clinical services must also be alert to the arrival of new knowledge that can increase value. In an ideal world, all clinicians would be motivated not only to adopt new (high-value) technology, but also to monitor new knowledge to identify evidence of higher-value interventions and of ineffective or lower-value interventions. Such evidence would lead clinicians to start stopping a service or longstanding clinical practice. In reality, people tend to be slow to adopt new knowledge, even knowledge that does not increase costs, such as the evidence that a checklist used prior to surgery reduces the risk of harm. (9) Clinicians may not start stopping long- established practices unless they are motivated to find the resources to fund an innovation that they want and which they believe will add value to the service.

In England, the National Institute for Health and Care Excellence (NICE) has made a major contribution to improving the management of innovation by the NHS, particularly where new drugs are concerned. New equipment and new procedures, such as new surgical operations, or new models of service delivery, such as a new screening programme, are more difficult to manage:

- *the research to assess their effectiveness is more difficult to undertake*
- *implementation is much more difficult, being dependent on the skill of the surgeon or the functioning of a multidisciplinary team, or both*

鼓励高价值创新，避免低价值创新

创新通常与启动新服务或新程序有关；但要管理好创新，另外两项活动更为重要：

- 停止启动（stopping starting）——即阻止低价值干预措施付诸实践。
- 启动停止（starting stopping）——即停止低价值的活动以便资源可以被释放出来重新使用，也被称为撤资。

临床服务管理者要谨慎使用不能增加价值的新技术，如已经使用，在低价值干预措施被叫停或缩减之前就应当提前引入能够增加价值的新技术。管控采购和订单可以评估新技术。但是，新技术有可能以各种方式绕过评估过程：

- 通过开发者租借给其他人；
- 伪装成研究项目；
- 在改变临床实践的尝试中，由制造商免费提供；
- 在改变临床实践的尝试中，被慈善机构收购。

临床服务管理者也必须对能够增加价值的新知识保持敏感性。在理想情况下，所有的临床医生不仅会主动采用新的（高价值的）技术，而且也会主动获取有关高价值的、无价值或低价值的干预措施证据的新知识。这些证据会引导临床医生叫停止某项服务或长期临床实践。即使是像"手术前使用检查表可以降低伤害风险"这类不会增加成本的知识，人们接受的速度仍然缓慢。临床医生可能不会叫停长期临床实践惯例，除非有动力鼓励他们去寻找资源进行他们想要的且相信会增加服务价值的创新。

在英国，国家卫生和保健优化研究所（NICE）为改善 NHS 的创新管理做出了重大贡献，尤其是在涉及新药的领域。新设备和新程序（如新外科术式）或提供服务的新模式（例如新的筛查方案）更难以管理，是因为：

- 评估其有效性的研究更加难以开展；
- 实施起来要困难得多，这要依赖于外科医生的技能或多学科团队的合作或两者兼而有之。

When compared with the management of innovation, it is more difficult to manage the drift to inappropriate and futile care. The phenomenon of drift was first described by David Eddy (10) as being one of three battles to watch in the 1990s. He highlighted that one of the main factors increasing healthcare costs was 'changes in the volume and intensity' of clinical practice. He argued that this apparently inexorable increase in the volume and intensity of clinical practice must be managed if increasingly scarce resources are to be used effectively.

When an evidence-based innovation is first introduced, it is provided to a group of patients who have characteristics similar to the characteristics of the patients in the original research study from which the evidence base was generated. Clinicians, however, often have to use their judgement in routine clinical practice because there are very few patients who are identical to the patients in the original research study. This is because the study design often stipulates entry criteria that are rarely encountered in clinical practice. For instance, the entry criteria for a heart-failure trial might be restricted to people with heart failure under 65 years of age who do not have any co-morbidities, whereas most patients with heart failure are over 65 years of age with co- morbidities. Thus, although clinicians may give the intervention to a tightly defined group of patients to begin with, over the years the intervention may be offered to other patients who have different indications or co-morbidities or who may be less severely affected.

Encouraging disinvestment from lower-value interventions

For the person managing a clinical service, there are several approaches to promoting disinvestment in lower-value interventions:

- *encouraging innovation within a fixed budget, thereby driving, and rewarding, the removal of lower-value work*
- *encouraging disinvestment directly, which requires a framework clinicians can use to identify lower-value activities (see Box 1.9)*

To maximise value, it is essential to manage both innovation and disinvestment; leaving the maximisation of value to natural evolution is a high-risk strategy unlikely to succeed, even though it is commonplace in an ever-expanding healthcare industry.

Box 1.9 Framework to identify lower-value activities

- As specialists, are we seeing patients who could be managed equally as well by general practitioners?
- Are there clinical activities for which there is no evidence of benefit that we could stop?
- Are there clinical activities for which there is no supporting evidence that we could stop or have a trial to investigate stopping?
- Can we identify waste, i.e. non-clinical activity that adds no value?

与创新管理相比，更难以实现的是扭转不当或无用的医疗卫生保健措施。这最初被大卫·埃迪认为是 20 世纪 90 年代三个值得关注的战役之一。他强调，增加医疗卫生保健成本的主要因素之一是临床实践中"数量和强度的变化"。他认为，如果要有效利用日益稀缺的资源，对明显且不可避免的临床实践在数量和强度的增加方面要加强管理。

当首次引入一项循证创新时，它被提供给一组特征与原始研究中特征相似的患者，从而产生了证据库。然而，由于很少有患者与原始研究中的患者完全相同，临床医生在日常临床实践中往往不得不自行判断。导致此项的原因是在原始研究设计中通常规定的纳入标准、在临床实践中很少遇到。例如，心力衰竭试验的纳入标准可能局限于 65 岁以下没有任何合并症的心力衰竭患者，而大多数心力衰竭患者是 65 岁以上有合并症的患者。因此，虽然临床医生一开始可能只对一组严格定义的患者进行干预，但多年以后，可能会对其他有不同适应证、合并症或较轻的患者进行干预。

鼓励从低价值干预中撤资

对于临床服务管理者来说，有几种方法可减少对低价值干预措施的投入：

- 在固定预算内鼓励创新，从而推动并奖励消除低价值工作；
- 鼓励直接撤资，这需要一个简要评估工具，临床医生可以使用它来识别那些低价值的活动（专栏 1.9）。

要实现价值最大化，必须同时管理创新并减少投资。将价值最大化留待于自然选择实现，是一种不太可能成功的高风险策略，尽管这在不断扩张的医疗卫生保健行业是常见策略。

专栏 1.9　用于识别低价值活动的框架

- 作为专科医生，我们所诊治的患者是否也可以在全科医生那里得到同等的治疗？
- 我们是否可以停止那些缺乏有益证据的临床活动？
- 对于没有得到证据支持的临床活动，我们是否可以停止或开展试验以使之停止？
- 我们能否识别浪费（如没有增加价值）的非临床活动？

Step 6: Getting the right outcome for the right patient

See page 50.

Step 7: Reducing waste

Refer to the following section 'Responsibility for reducing waste and increasing sustainability'.

■ Responsibility for reducing waste and increasing sustainability

> *Your waste denies me a service.*
>
> *User of Alaska Native health system*

As discussed above, value is determined by the relationship between outcome and the resources used. It is the responsibility of the clinician serving a particular population to minimise the amount of resources used. Minimising resource use contributes to increasing sustainability. In the context of sustainability, the use of the term resources does not refer to money alone.

The relationship between reducing waste and increasing sustainability is shown in Figure 1.26. The reduction of waste in health services has immediate benefits because it can release resources which are then available to treat more members of the population. Moreover, there are other longer-term benefits that result not only from reducing waste in healthcare but also from increasing the level of sustainability.

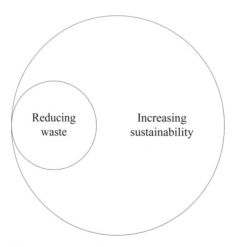

Figure 1.26   The relationship between waste and sustainability

To be a good steward of resources for the population, clinicians practising population medicine need to reduce waste and increase sustainability, and not simply to cut budgets. Clinicians must prevent the waste of time, the time of both clinicians and patients, and the unnecessary use of carbon.

第六步：让适合的患者能够得到正确的结局。

见第 1 章第 3 节 "使每一位患者都能得到正确的医疗结局"。

第七步：减少浪费

请参阅以下章节 "减少浪费与提高可持续性的责任"。

■ 减少浪费和提高可持续性的责任

> 你的浪费使我得不到医疗卫生保健。
>
> ——阿拉斯加的原住民卫生系统用户

如上所述，价值取决于结果和所用资源之间的关系。临床医生为特定人群服务时，有责任尽量减少资源的使用量。最小化的资源使用有助于提高可持续性。在可持续性的方面，资源的含义不仅仅包括金钱。

减少浪费和提高可持续性之间的关系如图 1.26 所示。减少医疗卫生保健中的浪费有立竿见影的收益，它可以释放医疗资源并用于治疗更多的人。此外，减少浪费不仅能够节约医疗卫生资源，还可以增加可持续性的程度，从而取得长远收益。

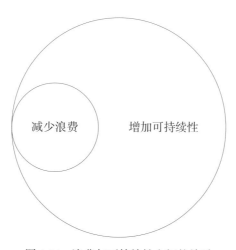

图 1.26　浪费与可持续性之间的关系

为了妥善管理人群现有的资源，从事群医学的医生不仅仅需要简单地削减预算，还需减少浪费并提高可持续性。临床医生必须避免浪费时间，无论是临床医生还是患者的时间，以及不必要的碳资源消耗。

Down with *muda*

In the absence of new resources, those who manage healthcare, many of whom are clinicians, must obtain greater value from the resources available in order to meet increasing need and demand. One way to obtain greater value is to reduce waste. In this situation, there is much to learn from Toyota's success, which is due to an obsession with:

- *kaizan, the relentless pursuit of better quality, and mass customisation (the analogue of personalised medicine)*
- *the eradication of muda, or waste, which Toyota define as ' … any activity, service, or supply that consumes time, money, and other resources, but creates no value.' (11)*

The Toyota formula, which can be applied to health services (12), is:

Work done = Work that produces value + Waste (11)

Taiichi Ohno, one of the driving forces behind Toyota, created the obsession with the eradication of muda. He identified seven categories of waste in industrial systems, which are relevant to healthcare:

1. Overproduction
2. Time on hand (waiting)
3. Stock on hand (inventory)
4. Waste of movement
5. Defective products
6. Transportation
7. Processing

Ohno's work, and the concept of 'lean thinking' (12) which flowed from it, are of central importance to those who pay for, or manage, health services. Indeed, Ohno's seven categories of waste have been adapted by Toussaint, Gerard and Womack (13) to apply to healthcare (see Box 1.10).

Box 1.10 Eight types of waste in healthcare (13)

- Defect: making errors, inspecting work already done for error
- Waiting: for test results to be delivered, for an appointment, for a bed, for a release of paperwork
- Motion: searching for supplies, fetching drugs from another room, looking for proper forms
- Transportation: taking patients through miles of corridors, from one test to the next unnecessarily, transferring patients to new rooms or units, carrying trays of tools between rooms

避免浪费

在缺乏新资源的情况下，从事医疗卫生保健的专业人员（其中许多是临床医生）必须从现有资源中获得更大的价值，以满足日益增长的卫生服务需求。获得更大价值的方法之一是减少浪费。在这种情况下，丰田的成功有很多值得学习的地方，其坚持的几点包括：

- 改善（Kaizan）——对更高质量的不懈追求和大规模定制服务（类似于个性化医疗）；
- 消除浪费，所谓"浪费"丰田将其定义为"……任何消耗时间、金钱和其他资源但没有创造价值的活动、服务或供应[11]。"
- 丰田公式可以应用于医疗卫生保健服务[12]，即：

$$已完成的工作 = 创造价值的工作 + 浪费^{[11]}$$

大野泰一是丰田幕后推手之一，他创造了消除浪费的理念。他提出了工业系统中的七个浪费类别，与医疗卫生保健具有共性：

1. 生产过剩；

2. 现有的时间（等待）；

3. 现有的库存（滞存）；

4. 运转过程的损耗；

5. 瑕疵品；

6. 交通运输；

7. 流程设置。

大野泰一的工作，以及由此产生的"精益思维"[12]的概念，对于卫生服务的支付者或管理者来说非常重要。事实上，大野太一的七类浪费已经被托桑、杰拉德和沃玛克[13]采纳并应用于医疗卫生保健领域（专栏1.10）。

专栏 1.10　医疗卫生保健中的八种浪费[13]

- **缺点**：错误已酿成，却再次检查导致错误的工作。
- **等待**：等待测试结果，等待预约、床位、文件公布。
- **行动**：寻找物资，从其他房间取药，寻找合适的单据。
- **转运**：带患者穿过数英里长的走廊，不必要地进行一个又一个检查，将患者转移到新的房间或单元，在房间之间搬运放工具的托盘。

continued

> • Defect: making errors, inspecting work already done for error
> • Waiting: for test results to be delivered, for an appointment, for a bed, for a release of paperwork
> • Motion: searching for supplies, fetching drugs from another room, looking for proper forms
> • Transportation: taking patients through miles of corridors, from one test to the next unnecessarily, transferring patients to new rooms or units, carrying trays of tools between rooms
> • Overproduction: excessive diagnostic testing, unnecessary treatment
> • Overprocessing: a patient being asked the same question three times, unnecessary forms, nurses writing everything in a chart instead of noting exceptions
> • Inventory: too much or too little; overstocked drugs expiring on the shelf, under-stocked surgical supplies delaying procedures while staff go in search of needed items
> • Talent: failing to listen to employee ideas for innovation

In an important article, Don Berwick estimated that the cost of waste 'exceeds 20% of total health care expenditure'. (14) The six types of waste he identified are:

- *Overtreatment*
- *Failures of care coordination*
- *Failures in execution of care processes*
- *Administrative complexity*
- *Pricing failures*
- *Fraud and abuse*

High-value population medicine involves getting the right patients to the right service and the right treatment done right first time. (When taking decisions about what is 'right', lower-value activities need to be identified and excluded.) It is also essential to identify and reduce waste, even when the right interventions are being delivered safely and at high quality to the right patients.

Clinicians responsible for serving a population need to minimise waste for two main reasons:

- *they have a responsibility to the population providing the resources for healthcare not to waste those resources, which could otherwise be spent on other public services such as education or social services*
- *to release resources so that more people in need in the population can be treated*

Eight questions to help clinicians identify and minimise waste are shown in Box 1.11.

续表

> - 生产过剩：过度诊断测试，不必要的治疗。
> - 过度处理：患者同一个问题被问了 3 次，填写不必要的表格，护士把所有的东西都写在图表上而非仅对异常情况进行记录。
> - 现有库存：太多或太少；库存货架上积压了过期的药品，当医务人员寻找所需的物品时，手术用品又库存不足，耽误了手术。
> - 人才：未能听取员工的创新想法。

　　唐·贝里克在一篇重要文章中估计，浪费的成本"超过了医疗卫生保健总开支的 20%"[14]。他确定的六类浪费是：

- 过度治疗；
- 医疗服务中的协作不足；
- 医疗服务过程中执行失误；
- 冗杂的行政管理；
- 定价不合理；
- 欺瞒和滥用。

　　高价值的群医学就是要让正确的患者获得正确的服务，并在正确的时间进行正确的治疗（当决定什么才算是"正确的"时，需要确定并排除那些低价值的活动）。确定和减少浪费也非常重要，即使是在安全高质量地向正确的患者提供正确的干预措施时也应如此。

　　为人群提供服务的临床医生需要减少浪费，主要有以下两个原因：

- 他们有责任为人群提供医疗卫生保健资源，且不应浪费，因为这些资源本来也可以用于其他公共服务，如教育或社会服务。
- 发放资源，使更多有需要的人都能够得到治疗。

帮助临床医生识别和减少浪费的八个问题，如专栏 1.11 所示。

Box 1.11 Questions to identify waste in health services (14)

- Can we make more use of buildings and equipment?
- Do we need to carry as much stock?
- Could care be provided by less highly-paid staff?
- Can the numbers of non-clinical staff be reduced?
- Can the waste of clinician and patient time be reduced?
- Is care being delivered in the right place?
- Can we use cheaper drugs and equipment?
- Can we prevent waste of human resources?

Question 1: Can we make more use of buildings and equipment?

In most countries, hospitals serve small populations of 100,000–300,000 people. In New Zealand, there are 20 District Health Boards covering a population of four million people.

This pattern of development was initiated in an era in when:

- *there was little specialisation other than that between medical and surgical specialties*
- *car ownership was low*
- *medical technology, such as imaging technology, was much simpler and less expensive than it is today*
- *the mobile 'phone had not even been imagined*

Today, we have a configuration of health services in which there are too many hospitals with under-utilised buildings and equipment. The considerable growth in the size of hospitals during the last 50 years has largely been characterised by development in isolation and development in competition – the 'medical arms race'. Not every hospital needs to provide every specialty and every piece of equipment. For hospitals to give up a specialty or to choose not to develop a specialty requires strong clinical leadership. Clinicians practising population medicine need to be able to demonstrate that it is in the best interests of the population served, to whom they are accountable, for some members of that population to have to travel further for certain services so that resources are not used in the unnecessary duplication of services.

Saving the resources entailed in duplication will enable a greater number of patients in need to be treated. Fortunately, this strategy is also often in the best interests of individual patients.

专栏 **1.11** **用于识别医疗卫生服务中的浪费问题**[14]

- 我们能否更充分地利用场所空间和设备器材？

- 我们需要多少库存？

- 医疗服务是否可以由薪酬稍低的员工们来提供？

- 能否减少非临床医务人员的数量？

- 能否减少对临床医生和患者时间的浪费？

- 是在正确的地方提供了医疗服务吗？

- 我们能否使用更便宜的药品和设备器材？

- 我们能否防止人力资源浪费？

问题 1：我们能否更充分地利用场所空间和设备器材？

在大多数国家，医院为 10 万至 30 万人的小规模人群提供服务。在新西兰，20 个地区的卫生局覆盖了 400 万人口。

这种发展模式始于这个时代：

- 除了内科和外科专业之外，几乎没有其他专科；

- 有车的人很少；

- 医疗技术，如成像技术，比现在简单得多，也便宜得多；

- 移动电话尚未问世。

目前，在我们的医疗卫生保健卫生服务配置中，有太多医院的场所空间和设备器材利用不足。在过去 50 年中，医院规模的显著增长主要表现是在孤立中发展和在竞争中发展，即"医疗军备竞赛"。不是每一家医院都需要提供每一种专科和每一种设备。对于医院来说，放弃某项专科或选择不发展某个专科，都需要有具备强大的临床领导才能。从事群医学的临床医生应该有能力向所服务的人群说明：为了保证群体利益最大化，一些人需要前往其他医疗机构获得特定的医疗服务，以避免因为不必要的重复服务而过度使用资源。

节省重复性工作中的资源将使更多需要治疗的患者能够得到救治。幸运的是，这种策略通常也符合患者个人的最大利益。

Question 2: Do we need to carry as much stock?

In 2005, 574 different head and socket combinations were used in [hip replacement] operations in England and Wales. It seems implausible that meaningful data can be gathered, or that money can be saved through bulk purchase, when such a number of products and supplies is used in this way. (15)

Just-in-time delivery of the equipment needed was one of the great achievements of the Toyota production systems, and provides much useful learning for health services. In contrast, most health services buy too much equipment of too many types and store it for too long.

Such waste can be prevented partly by improving procurement practices, but staff responsible for procurement do not act in isolation. They tend to buy what clinicians want, seeking the lowest possible price but not necessarily questioning the added value of the new item that a clinician has requested.

Rather, the rigorous appraisal of requests relating to clinical procurement should be done by the clinician leading on population medicine. This clinician must persuade colleagues that it is not only the cost of new medical devices that wastes resources, but also the costs of storage, stock control and the disposal of unused or unwanted devices. Here, pharmacies represent a model of good stock control that other hospital departments can follow.

Question 3: Could care be provided by less highly paid staff?

Highly trained staff are scarce and expensive to train. It is a waste of skill if highly trained staff undertake tasks that could be managed equally well by other staff who have not had the same level of skills development but whose training has enabled them to carry out a specific range of tasks. Less highly trained staff are able not only to undertake repetitive tasks with greater attention to detail but also to obtain better results than those achieved by the most highly trained staff for whom such tasks are not relevant to their core function.

Question 4: Can the numbers of non-clinical staff be reduced?

Contrary to popular belief, administrative staff do not create their own work.

- *The work of staff in the central management of a health service is created by outside agencies, which impose certain tasks or require specific information on a regular basis*
- *Much of the work of administrative staff in clinical areas is created by clinicians; some of the administrative tasks may be unnecessary tasks but only because clinicians have not addressed the need to make the work of 'clinical microsystems' leaner*

问题 2：我们需要多少库存？

2005 年，英格兰和威尔士的（髋关节置换）手术中使用了 574 种不同的头窝组合。当使用了如此多的产品和用品时，想要收集有意义的数据或通过批量采购节省开支是不切实际的[15]。

能够及时交付所需设备器材是丰田生产系统的一大成绩，为医疗卫生保健服务提供了许多有益借鉴。相比之下，大多数医疗卫生保健服务购买了过多种类的设备器材，并且闲置时间过长。

通过改进采购方法可以在一定程度上防止这种浪费，但负责采购的工作人员不应独自行动。他们虽倾向于购买临床医生想要的东西，并寻求可能的最低价格，但不一定会质疑临床医生所要求新产品的附加值。相反，应该由群医学领域的临床医生来严格评估与临床采购相关的申请。

该临床医生必须说服同事们认识到：资源的浪费不仅存在于购买新医疗器械的花费，还存在于存储、控制库存以及处理未使用或不需要设备的成本等方面。在此，药房展现了一种良好的库存控制模式，医院的其他部门可以效仿。

问题 3：是否可以让薪酬较低员工来提供医疗服务？

训练有素的医务人员人数稀少且培训成本高。如果他们所承担的工作本可在确保质量的同时由未经高级培训人员开展，会造成一种技术上的浪费。这些接受培训较少的医务人员即便没有接受足够完备的培训，仍能完成一些特定任务，他们虽受过的高级培训较少，但在重复性工作中会更加注重细节，而且能把工作做得比受高级培训的医务人员更好。也因为这些任务往往并不是接受过高级培训的医务人员的核心职务。

问题 4：能否减少非临床医务人员数量？

与大众认识不同的是，行政管理人员并不能自己创建工作内容。

- 只有当某些外部机构需要定期开展某些工作或需要某些具体信息时，才有了医疗卫生保健核心管理工作人员的工作任务。
- 临床管理人员的大部分工作是由临床医生提出的；某些管理任务可能是不必要的，只是由于临床医生尚未能精简"临床微系统"的工作。

A clinical microsystem is a small group of people who work together on a regular basis to provide care to discrete subpopulations of patients. It has clinical and business aims, linked processes, and a shared information environment, and it produces performance outcomes. (16)

Even teams that work well together may undertake lower-value activities that have crept into their clinical practice over the years, and which need to be eradicated, such as:

- *collecting data that no-one uses (or which are used inappropriately)*
- *handovers done on paper that could be done digitally*

Lower-value activities lead to a failure to incorporate higher-value activities, such as involving the patient as a key member of the team.

Question 5: Can the waste of clinician and patient time be reduced?

For clinicians, time is the scarcest resource: it is finite and once expended cannot be recovered. Unfortunately, much of a clinician's time is wasted. Often, the job of a clinician involves more than encounters with patients during clinical practice. It can encompass management, education and research. All these aspects of a clinician's job, including clinical practice, while intrinsically valuable, can incur a waste of time.

Waste of time in management

Many clinicians are reimbursed for half a day in recognition of the time spent in managing resources, but much of this can be considered a 'waste', undertaking activities such as:

- *writing a plan that has no possibility of realisation*
- *contributing to projects that are poorly managed or do not deliver the anticipated outputs*
- *meetings without purpose or conclusion*

All clinicians are more than likely to have their own ideas about what constitutes a waste of time, but their perceptions may not be shared. Attendance at a management meeting may be considered a waste of time by a clinician, but regarded as of high value by a manager. Independent evaluation is required to determine which of the two perceptions is correct: the clinician because the meeting was unfocused and unproductive, or the manager because the clinician attended a meeting that was of value but the clinician approached it with an unhelpful attitude.

所谓的临床微系统是指：一小群人定期地共同为离群、散居的患者提供医疗卫生保健。该系统有临床和业务目标、相互关联的流程和共享的信息环境，并产生绩效结果[16]。

即使是合作良好的团队，也可能会从事一些低价值的活动。这些低价值活动已在过去的几年里渗透到了临床实践中，有待根除，例如：

- 收集无人使用（或使用不当）的数据；
- 仍采用纸质交接可数字化的工作。

价值较低的活动导致了它们与价值较高的活动相整合，如让患者成为团队的关键成员。

问题5：能否减少临床医生和患者在时间上的浪费？

对临床医生来说时间是最稀缺的资源：时间是有限的，且一旦被使用就无法再生。不幸的是，临床医生的许多时间都被浪费了。通常，临床医生的工作不仅仅是在临床工作中治疗患者，还包括管理、教育和科学研究工作。临床医生的这些工作，包括临床实践，虽然本质上是有价值的，但都可能导致时间的浪费。

在管理中浪费的时间

考虑到在管理资源上花费的时间，许多临床医生可以得到半天的补偿。但如从事以下活动时，这"半天的补偿"也可以被视为是"浪费"。这些活动包括：

- 编写不可能实现的计划；
- 参与管理不善或无法交付预期成果的项目；
- 参加无目的或无结论的会议。

临床医生对什么是浪费时间很可能有自己的认识，但看法不一定一致。临床医生可能会认为参加管理会议是在浪费时间，但管理者却认为会议很有价值。临床医生认为会议没有重点也没有产出；管理者认为临床医生参加的会议有其价值所在，但参会医生态度敷衍了事（因此无法从中有所获益），这两种观点哪一种正确，需要分别从不同角度独立评估分析。

Waste of time in education

Education can have benefits, but it is always associated with a cost. Education is of low value or represents a waste of time if:

- *the intervention has been selected in accordance with the clinician's desire rather than through a formal assessment of learning needs (there is evidence that if clinicians are interested in a topic, they will seek the learning they need) (17)*
- *the educational methods used are not supported by evidence of effectiveness (for example, lectures are usually of low value)*

Waste of time in research

The value of investing public money in research is hotly debated, but most countries in Europe and North America now realise that it is important to develop an economy based on knowledge rather than one based on exporting agricultural products or manufactured goods.

Much could be done to increase the level of productivity and reduce the level of waste in research. (18) Specifically, Chalmers and Glasziou identified waste at all four stages of the research process (see Box 1.12).

Box 1.12 Avoidable waste in the clinical research process (18)

- Choosing the wrong question for research
- Doing studies that are unnecessary or poorly designed
- Failing to publish results promptly or not at all
- Producing biased or unusable reports of research

Waste of time in clinical practice

Clinical practice is of high value, but within the course of clinical work time is wasted if:

- *the patient's notes are missing*
- *key data, such as laboratory results, are not available*
- *there is unnecessary waiting time, such as between operations in theatre*

Wasting the time of patients

The problems that waste the time of clinicians can also waste the time of

在教学中浪费的时间

教育可以带来效益，但总与成本有关。教学在下列情况可视为价值很低或是浪费时间：

- 学习内容是根据临床医生的主观意愿而不是通过对学习需求的正式评估来选择的（有证据表明，如果临床医生对某个主题感兴趣，他们就会根据自己的需求学习）[17]。
- 没有证据可证明所使用的教育方法是有效的（例如，讲座的价值通常很低）。

在研究中浪费的时间

将公共资金投资于研究一直饱受争议，但欧洲和北美的大多数国家现在都意识到，经济发展靠的是知识，而非出口农产品或工业成品。

在提高生产力水平和减少研究中的浪费方面有很多工作可以做[18]。具体而言，Chalmers 和 Glasziou 发现在研究过程的四个阶段都可能产生浪费（专栏 1.12）。

专栏 1.12 临床研究过程中可避免的浪费[18]

- 选择错误的研究问题。
- 进行不必要或设计不当的研究项目。
- 未能及时或根本不发表其研究结果。
- 得出有偏倚的或无用的研究报告。

在临床实践中浪费时间

临床实践是有很高价值的。但在临床工作过程中，如果有以下情况则是在浪费时间：

- 缺失了患者的有关记录；
- 无法获取关键数据，如实验室结果；
- 不必要的等待时间，如手术室中两次手术之间的等待时间。

浪费患者的时间

浪费临床医生时间的问题同样会浪费患者时间，特别是当人们越来越认

patients, especially as there is increasing recognition that patients need to make a considerable contribution to their own care even if they do not have to pay for the cost of it. The concept of a 'treatment burden' draws attention to the four types of 'work' that patients with complex problems have to undertake (see Box 1.13). Considering the burden of work for patients receiving care, it is important that clinicians and other healthcare professionals give careful consideration to the ways in which patients' time is wasted and how this may be ameliorated.

Box 1.13 Work undertaken by patients with complex problems during treatment (19)

- Learning about treatments and their consequences: sensemaking work
- Engaging with others/mobilizing resources: participation work
- Adhering to treatments and lifestyle changes: enacting work
- Monitoring the treatments: appraisal work

Question 6: Is care being delivered in the right place?

Many patients receive care at healthcare facilities where the levels of staffing and other resources are of an intensity unnecessary for good patient outcomes. Patients who are usually cared for in secondary care facility but could be cared for elsewhere include:

- *patients, usually older people, who have recovered from the acute phase of their disease but cannot be discharged because they are too disabled to return home to a supported environment and yet cannot be found a place in a nursing home. This situation is of concern not only for those who manage or pay for care but also for the patients who are at high risk of hospital-acquired infection, institutionalisation, and malnutrition*
- *patients who attend a clinic with a problem that could have been resolved if their primary care clinician had had a convenient and fast method of accessing the expertise of the specialist, such as via an email, a 'phone call or a video link*
- *people who die in hospital who could have been supported to die at home*

Question 7: Can we use cheaper equipment and drugs?

The key question when considering waste in relation to equipment and drugs is why pay more than is necessary? Costs can be reduced by:

- *skilful procurement*
- *bulk purchase*
- *the use of generic rather than branded drugs (with significant savings as illustrated in New Zealand by the highly successful PHARMAC)*

识到，即便患者不必支付任何费用，他们还是需要为自己的医疗卫生保健护理做出很多贡献。"治疗的负担"这一概念使人们注意到具有复合型问题的患者自身必须承担的四种"工作"（专栏 1.13）。考虑到照护患者的工作负担，临床医生和其他医疗卫生专业人员应仔细考虑患者的时间是以什么方式被浪费的以及如何改进。

专栏 1.13　具有复合型问题的患者在治疗期间需要做的事情[19]

- 了解治疗及其后果：感知。
- 与他人交流 / 筹集资源：参与。
- 坚持治疗和改变生活方式：配合。
- 监测治疗：评估。

问题 6：是否在正确的地点提供了医疗卫生保健？

许多患者在医疗机构接受医疗卫生保健，但该机构中配备人员和资源级别对于患者的良好预后完全没有必要。通常患者在二级卫生保健机构接受的医疗卫生保健也同样可以在其他地方得到，包括：

- 已经从疾病急性期恢复、但由于行动不便无法居家疗养却又找不到康复疗养机构而不能出院的患者，尤其是老年人。这种情况不仅关系到那些管理或支付费用的人，也关系到那些可有较高风险发生院内感染、长期住在养老机构和发生营养不良的患者。

- 到诊所就诊的患者的问题可以通过下述方式得到解决：患者的初级卫生保健医生能通过电子邮件、电话或视频等方便快捷的方式、从专科医学处获得相关的专业知识。

- 本可以在家中接受临终关怀的患者却在医院里去世。

问题 7：我们能否使用更便宜的药品和设备器材？

在考虑与设备和药品有关的浪费时，关键问题是为什么要支付更多不必要的费用？以下方式可以降低成本：

- 有技巧地采购；

- 成批量付款；

- 使用仿制药而非品牌药品（在新西兰取得巨大成功的制药公司 PHARMAC 证明了这一点）；

- *'making' rather than 'buying'*
- *sharing services*

These activities are ethically important because they reduce waste, increase productivity and release resources for clinical care.

Alternatives to interventions often exist, and once cost–benefit or cost–utility analysis has been used to assess whether an intervention offers good value, cost-effectiveness analysis enables a comparison of two or more methods of achieving the desired result. The aim of cost-effectiveness analysis is to identify the lowest cost option.

> *... [cost-effectiveness analysis] compares the costs of alternative ways of achieving a given objective. Where two or more interventions are found to achieve the same level of benefits, the intervention with the least cost is the most cost-effective alternative. (20)*

- *If cost–benefit analysis demonstrates the value of revascularisation of the coronary arteries, cost–effectiveness analysis enables two methods, coronary artery bypass grafting and stenting, to be compared*
- *If cost–benefit analysis demonstrates that the treatment of less severe depression appears to have benefit, cost–effectiveness analysis can be used to answer the question of whether it is less costly to use drugs or cognitive therapy*

Thus, the clinician can choose the intervention that is more cost-effective.

Irrespective of the answer to questions posed during cost–effectiveness analysis, there is a supplementary question concerning costliness, for example:

- *Which drug is the least costly?*
- *Is face-to-face or online consultation less costly?*

Such questions are often more subtle and less clear-cut than would appear at first sight. There may be small differences in the magnitude of the benefits and harms of each option, or in the probabilities of good and bad outcomes. The decisions about which of the options to choose involve not only a cost comparison but also a judgement about which of the trade-offs associated with each option is preferred in the current context. The simplest type of comparison is that regarding the use of a generic drug when compared with the proprietary product because both interventions are identical in effect but different in price; clinicians do not always choose the cheapest option in this situation.

- "制造"而非"购买";

- 共享医疗卫生保健。

这些行动减少了浪费，提高了生产力，并为临床治疗护理提供了资源，从伦理角度看非常重要。

干预措施通常存在有可替代的方法而使用成本 – 效益分析或成本 – 效用可用来分析来评估干预措施是否具有良好价值，成本 – 效果分析就可以对两种或更多种干预措施进行比较，看哪一种方法更可达到预期的结果。成本 – 效果分析的目的是确定最低成本的选择。

> ……[成本 – 效果分析] 比较了实现既定目标的各种备选方案的成本。如果发现两种或两种以上的干预措施能够获得相同的效益水平，则成本最低的干预措施是最具成本 – 效果的替代方案[20]。

- 如果成本 – 效益分析可以证明冠状动脉血运重建的价值，那么成本 – 效果分析就可以比较冠状动脉搭桥术和支架置入术这两种方法。

- 如果成本 – 效益分析表明，治疗轻度抑郁症获得的效益更高，那么成本 – 效果分析可以用来回答下述问题：在药物或认知疗法二者间，哪种方法成本更低。

因此，临床医生可以选择更具成本 – 效果的干预措施。

无论成本 – 效益分析期间所提问题的答案是什么，都有一个关于成本的补充问题，例如：

- 哪种药最便宜?

- 面对面咨询和在线咨询，哪一种的成本更低?

这类问题往往比乍看上去更微妙也更模糊。每种选择的利弊或结果好坏上可能仅有微小差别。决定选择哪种方案不仅涉及其成本比较，还需权衡每个选项的交互关系，才能做出当下最适宜的选择。最简单的比较方式是把常用药与专利产品相比，因为两种药物的干预效果相同而价格相异；而在这种情况下，临床医生并不一定总会选择那些最便宜的。

Question 8: Can we prevent waste of human resources?

Demanding though it may be to work on the Toyota production line, that task is much simpler than those associated with clinical practice. For many people, the admonition not to waste the untapped potential of professionals would be interpreted as a call to provide more and better quality continuing professional development. The reality is that greater challenges face us:

- *staff retention and turnover – investment in training does not realise much value if a high proportion of those trained, such as nurses, leave within five years*
- *burnout – the largest waste of professional talent, particularly when considering the case of clinicians*

Burnout is usually identified by three major symptoms: emotional exhaustion, depersonalisation, and decreased sense of self-efficacy. But burnout, we believe is also a euphemism for what many physicians experience as a crisis of meaning and identity.

Burnout is the index of dislocation between what people are and what they have to do. It represents an erosion in values, dignity, spirit, and will – and erosion of the human soul. (21)

The main concern about burnout is not necessarily the loss of workforce and the waste of resources involved in workforce training, but that healthcare professionals can begin to work in a way that is detrimental to the service, annoying for colleagues and upsetting for any patients they may encounter. As pressure increases to meet rising need and demand in a context of no new resources while also continuing to improve quality and safety, in the absence of good leadership, the prevalence of burnout will increase. Indeed, the prevalence of burnout may be worsened by the need for managers to impose what has been called 'the target culture'. The impact of burnout in the USA could be serious, especially in the context of implementing universal coverage (22), but it is by no means a problem unique to the USA.

Even when burnout is not a problem experienced by clinicians and other healthcare professionals, staff can behave in other ways that are counter-productive and difficult to deal with such as the subtle withdrawal of enthusiasm. In developing a health service for a population, although it is essential to be concerned about strategy and systems, it is equally important to consider and empathise with the situation of frontline staff, and build appropriate support and development programmes to maintain the resilience of individuals and the workforce.

问题 8：我们能否防止人力资源的浪费？

虽然在丰田生产线上可能对工作要求很高，但比起临床实践相关的任务来说要简单得多。对很多人来说，不要浪费专业人才潜力的呼吁可以被解读为呼吁提供更多和更高质量的持续专业发展。但现实是我们正面临着更大的挑战：

- 医务人员的留用率和离职率——如果大部分受培训人员（如护士）在五年内离职，用于培训的投资就没有得到回报。
- 职业倦怠——这是对专业人才的最大浪费，尤其是临床医生。

职业倦怠通常有三个主要症状：情绪疲惫、人格解体和自我效能感下降。但是，我们相信它也是许多医生都经历的"人生意义和自我认同危机"的委婉说法。

职业倦怠显示了"我是谁，我该做什么"二者之间的混乱。它代表着对人类价值观、尊严、精神和意志等方面受到的侵蚀——以及对灵魂的侵蚀[21]。

职业倦怠的主要问题不一定是劳动力流失和职业培训的资源浪费，而是医护人员开始以一种不良方式工作，不仅使同事感到恼火也让被服务的患者感到失望。在没有新资源的情况下，持续改进质量和安全性以满足不断增长的卫生服务需要和需求，会导致压力不断增加；同时在没有良好领导的情况下，职业倦怠将更加普遍。确切来说，由于管理者强制实行所谓的"目标文化"，普遍性职业的倦怠可能会进一步恶化。美国职业倦怠的影响可能很严重，尤其是在实施全民医保的情况下[22]，但此问题绝非美国独有。

即使临床医生和其他医疗卫生专业人员没有遇到职业倦怠问题，员工也会以其他形式表现出逆反或难以应对的行为，如难以觉察到的工作热情降低等。在为某人群订制医疗卫生保健服务项目时，虽然策略和体系非常重要，但是也应该考虑和理解那些一线工作人员的状况、给予其适当的支持和改进项目的安排以保障个人和员工的承受力。这些措施也同样重要。

Reducing waste contributes to increased sustainability

Sustainability is a key concept for the 21st century, and the reduction of waste increases the sustainability of any organisation. Sustainability, however, covers a greater range of topics than the reduction of waste, and it is of central importance to population medicine. Healthcare in general also needs to become much more sustainable. (23)

The clinician fulfilling responsibilities for population medicine needs to consider the impact of clinical practice on the environment and not just the amount of resources consumed. The change in culture necessary to make sustainability a central concern, and not one at the margins, is one of the most important responsibilities in population medicine. Clinicians who manage healthcare need:

- *to reduce the carbon footprint of their services*
- *to increase the overall sustainability of their services*

In the UK, the renal service has set the standard for establishing sustainability as a central concern in clinical practice. (24)

The meaning of 'sustainable development'

The term 'sustainable development' is widely used and has different meanings for different people. Originally, the term was taken to have an environmental meaning, such as that shown in Box 1.14, but subsequently sustainable development was described as 'protecting resources from one generation to the next'. (25)

Box 1.14 The environmental meaning of sustainable development (26)

- Consuming fewer material goods
- Using locally produced goods and services to reduce their carbon emissions from their transportation – this will also contribute to the economic sustainability of local communities
- Ensuring that goods and services are produced in as energy-efficient a way as possible with minimal waste (which is recycled)
- Ensuring material goods (such as washing machines, TVs, fridges, etc.) are themselves energy efficient

The term, however, now has a broader meaning, perhaps best expressed in the following quotation from The Lancet's Global Health Commission:

> *The concept of sustainable development was formulated to address issues of intergenerational equity in resource availability. It has been condemned as lacking definition and conceptual rigour.*

减少浪费有助于提高可持续性

可持续发展是 21 世纪的重要概念，任何组织减少浪费均可提高可持续性。然而除了减少浪费，可持续性涵盖主题范围更广阔，并且这对群医学至关重要。一般而言，医疗卫生保健服务也需要提高可持续性[23]。

承担群医学职责的临床医生需要考虑临床实践对环境的影响，而不仅仅是资源的消耗量。进行必要的文化建设，使可持续发展成为核心而不是边缘内容，这是群医学最重要的职责之一。临床医生在从事医疗卫生保健的管理工作时，需要做到以下几点：

- 减少其服务的碳足迹。
- 提高其服务的整体可持续性。

在英国，肾脏服务中心已经制定了标准，将可持续性作为临床实践的核心问题[24]。

"可持续发展"的含义

"可持续发展"一词被广泛使用，并且不同的人有不同的理解。最初，这个词被认为有环境方面的含义，如专栏 1.14 所示，但后来指的是"保护后代资源"[25]。

专栏 1.14　可持续发展的环境含义[26]

- 减少物资消耗；
- 利用当地生产的商品和提供的服务，减少交通运输带来的碳排放，这也有助于当地经济的可持续发展；
- 确保生产产品和提供服务时，尽可能节约能源、减少浪费（回收利用）；
- 确保物资（如洗衣机、电视机、冰箱等）本身是节能的。

然而，这个词现在有了更广泛的含义，以下《柳叶刀》全球健康委员会的引文或许最能表达这一点：

> 提出可持续发展的概念是为了解决资源可及性的代际公平问题。它被责难缺乏定义和概念上的严谨性。

However, it offers the possibility of fundamental changes to the way we consume and produce, the way we arrange our functionally fragmented institutions, and the way we distribute resources globally and locally. Most importantly, sustainable development not only posits environmental degradation and poverty as interconnected issues, but it gives an example of how mainstream politics might be brought into a debate that demands a complete rethink of our institutions, resources, and environmental outcome, and also assumes that these issues can be solved with political will. (27)

Although sustainability now encompasses many issues, carbon and its effect on climate change are of vital concern to healthcare professionals because climate change is one of the principal threats to global health in the 21st century. This may be the reason why this issue tends to have the greatest potential for motivating frontline staff. Introducing a concern for sustainability can be encapsulated within a carbon reduction strategy.

Staff should have access to a range of materials highlighting the short- and long-term benefits of carbon reduction. Organisations must aspire to meet the targets established by national or international authorities and should communicate to staff that by meeting those targets many health and financial co-benefits will also be realised.

Reducing the carbon footprint of healthcare

The drive to increase value was described earlier in terms of being able to release resources for reallocation to meet some other need. This presupposes that the only relevant currency is money, whereas another important currency is carbon.

All healthcare organisations both public and private are expected to reduce their carbon footprint. In the United Kingdom, the NHS is the largest public sector contributor to climate change through its carbon emissions (23) – 21 million tonnes of CO_2 equivalents (MtCO_2e) in 2007. (28) The main sources contributing to NHS England's carbon footprint are shown in Figure 1.27.

Figure 1.27 illustrates why the emphasis in the White Paper Equity and Excellence: Liberating the NHS (29) on reducing the NHS' carbon footprint is not limited to decreasing energy used in the health service. To achieve significant overall reductions in carbon emissions will require clinicians to change the way in which they deliver care.

然而，它为我们在消费和生产的方式、在安排职能分散的机构以及在全球和地方如何分配资源的方式等方面都提供了根本性改变的可能。最重要的是，可持续发展不仅将环境退化和贫困视为相互关联的问题，而且还提供了一个实例，说明如何将主流政治也纳入对我们的体制，资源和环境结果进行全面反思的辩论并假设这些问题是可以通过政治意愿来解决的[27]。

尽管目前可持续性包含许多问题，但"碳及其对气候变化的影响"是医疗卫生专业人员极为关注的问题，因为气候变化是 21 世纪全球健康的主要威胁之一。这也许就是为什么这个问题最有可能调动那些在一线工作的员工积极性的原因。对可持续性的关注可以包含在碳减排的战略中。

工作人员应有机会接触到"强调减少碳排放的短期和长期效益"的一系列资料。各组织必须立志实现国家或国际社会制定的目标、并应与职员们沟通。通过实现这些目标，就可以实现健康和经济诸多方面的共赢。

减少医疗卫生保健的碳足迹

前面描述了增加价值的驱动力，即为满足更多需求，该如何释放资源并进行重新分配。此前提假设是："钱"是其唯一相关的硬通货，而另一个重要硬通货则是"碳"。

所有公共和私人医疗卫生保健机构都应该减少碳排放量。英国国家医疗服务体系（NHS）是通过碳排放而对气候变化影响最大的公共部门，其碳排放在 2007 年达到 2100 万吨二氧化碳当量（$MtCO_2e$）[28]。英国 NHS 碳排放量的主要来源如图 1.27 所示。

图 1.27 说明了《公平和卓越：解放英国 NHS 白皮书》[29] 所强调的减少 NHS 碳排放量并不局限于减少医疗卫生保健服务的能源使用。为了实现全面大幅减少碳排放，需要改变临床医生提供医疗服务的方式。

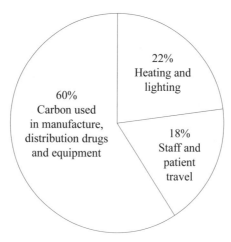

Figure 1.27   Sources contributing to the carbon footprint of NHS England (23)

Sustainable clinical practice

To reduce the carbon footprint of a healthcare service substantially requires a change in the style of clinical practice. Frances Mortimer, Medical Director of the Centre for Sustainable Healthcare in the United Kingdom, has developed a model of sustainable clinical practice (see Box 1.15).

Box 1.15 Model of sustainable clinical practice (30)

- All clinicians should be involved in prevention, the most sustainable type of health service
- Patient-centred care, for example, sending most laboratory results directly to patients to reduce the number of trips to health centres to collect results
- Leaner pathways, reducing the number of outpatient and follow-up appointments of low or no value
- The consideration of carbon costs as well as financial costs when considering the cost-effectiveness of treatment

Engaging staff in sustainability

Attitudes towards sustainability, and how to address it within a health service, vary. For some healthcare professionals, carbon reduction is an important issue because of concern about their children's future, but others may not be concerned that climate change is happening. Some staff believe that the health service, or their own part of the health service, is too small to make a difference. Suggestions about the ways in which to motivate staff to increase the sustainability of a health service are shown in Box 1.16.

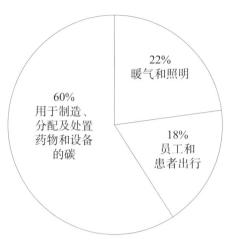

图 1.27 英国 NHS 碳排放量的来源[23]

可持续的临床实践

要减少医疗卫生保健服务的碳排放量，实质上需要改变临床实践的方式。英国可持续医疗中心主任弗朗西斯·莫蒂默开创了一种可持续的临床实践模式（专栏 1.15）。

专栏 1.15　可持续临床实践模式[30]

- 所有临床医生都应致力于预防，这是最具可持续性的医疗卫生保健服务类型。

- 以患者为中心的医疗服务，例如，将大多数实验室结果直接发送给患者，以减少前往医疗中心拿取结果的次数。

- 精简路径，减少低价值或无价值的门诊和随访预约数量。

- 在考虑治疗的成本 – 效果时也要考虑碳成本和经济成本。

让员工参与可持续发展

对可持续性的态度以及如何在医疗卫生保健服务中解决可持续性问题，众说纷纭。对于某些卫生医疗卫生保健服务界的专业人士来说，碳减排是一个重要问题，因为这关乎孩子的未来；但其他人可能对正在发生的气候变化并不在意。一些员工认为，医疗卫生保健服务或其自身所从事的卫生服务，由于影响范围太小而很难发挥作用。关于如何激励员工提高卫生服务可持续性的建议，见专栏 1.16。

Box 1.16 Ways to motivate staff to increase the sustainability of a health service

- Provide information about the effects of climate change on health
- Describe the factors that contribute to the carbon footprint of a health service
- Ask staff to report what their children are saying about climate change
- Ask how staff are changing their lifestyle to cope with either the threat of climate change or simply the rising cost of energy
- Introduce the concept of 'lean' production, namely, production without waste (some staff will be motivated by this whatever their views on climate change)
- Take part in projects to improve the natural environment of healthcare facilities

Another way of motivating staff is to provide financial and other incentives. Although It may be difficult to identify all the changes resulting from the implementation of a carbon reduction plan because, for example, the electricity used by the ward cannot be identified separately within a hospital's bill, it is usually possible to identify some measures to monitor the decreased use of resources. If carbon savings by a ward or health centre result in some financial reward, so much the better, but it is also important to appeal to the altruism of staff, encouraging them to take action for the good of society, and the next and future generations including their own children.

Adopting a broad approach to sustainability

It is important to adopt a broad approach to sustainability, considering such aspects as:

- *energy and carbon management*
- *procurement and food*
- *travel, transport and access*
- *water*
- *waste*
- *the built environment*
- *organisational and workforce development*
- *partnership and networks*
- *governance*
- *finance*

Organisation and workforce development

Imagine you are the director of a maternity service serving a deprived, multi-ethnic population. How would you recruit midwives? One approach is to advertise as widely as your budget allows with the aim of recruiting 'the best', but there are other approaches:

专栏 1.16　激励员工提高医疗卫生保健服务可持续性的方法

- 提供气候变化对健康影响的相关信息。
- 描述影响医疗服务碳排放量的各种因素。
- 请员工就自己孩子对气候变化的看法进行汇报。
- 询问员工如何改变生活方式以应对气候变化的威胁或仅是能源成本的上升（家庭开支的增加）等问题。
- 引入精益生产的概念，即无浪费生产（无论员工对气候变化的看法如何，某些员工都会为此受到激励）。
- 参与改善医疗卫生设施自然环境的项目。

激励员工的另一种方式是提供经济和其他方面的激励措施。尽管很难判断由于实施碳减排计划而产生的效果，例如，在医院的账单中无法单独确定病房所消耗的电能，但通常可以采取一些措施来监测资源的利用减少了多少。如果一个病房或健康中心的碳排放下降能带来一些经济回报，那就更好了。但同样重要的是呼吁员工的利他主义，鼓励他们为社会、包括子孙后代做出贡献。

采取广泛的可持续性方法

采取广泛的可持续性做法十分重要，考虑以下几个方面：

- 能源和碳管理；
- 采购和食品；
- 旅行、运输和使用；
- 水；
- 废弃物；
- 已建立起来的环境；
- 组织和劳动力发展；
- 合作关系和合作网络；
- 治理；
- 财政。

组织和劳动力的发展

想象一下，你是一家为贫困的少数族裔人群服务的妇产医疗机构的主管。你将如何招聘助产士？一种方法是在预算允许的范围内尽可能广泛地发布广告，目的是招聘"最优人选"。但也有其他方法：

- *avoid depleting the midwifery workforces of countries with developing economies as a matter of principle*
- *develop a programme in which midwives visit local primary and secondary schools and encourage girls in the surrounding communities to consider midwifery as a career*

Finance

Imagine you are a clinical director facing cuts to your budget. One approach is to reduce the costs of support services by outsourcing cleaning and secretarial services. This will reduce your financial costs but at the expense of the income of people who are already the lowest paid in the health service.

Another approach is to establish stronger links with the surrounding communities, encouraging the recruitment of local people who are more likely to develop a commitment to the local service and fulfil their responsibilities assiduously irrespective of the level of their salary.

Local sourcing, and not outsourcing, can be applied to other aspects of running a health service. Clinicians could consider promoting the procurement of food from the local foodshed (usually defined as food grown or sourced within a 50-km radius of the facility). Apart from the environmental benefits of reducing 'food miles' and thereby reducing carbon emissions, food sourced locally helps to retain money in the local economy and create wealth in the population served.

The realisation of sustainable development requires long-term planning, which takes into account not only the specific issues relating to healthcare facilities but also factors that could influence the determinants of health.

Although addressing the health service's impact on the determinants of health requires a much wider scope than that currently taken by many people who manage healthcare, this type of approach is now recognised as necessary.

> *For further thoughts on effective systems see Creating Systems (Book 1) in our Healthcare Transformation series.*

■ Questions for reflection

- *What is the best way to explain value to members of the public meeting to consider the budget of a health service?*
- *When looking for greater value, should the focus be on marginal analysis or on the main budget for a programme?*
- *How can clinicians be best encouraged to disinvest?*
- *What steps could be taken to reduce inappropriate and futile care?*
- *Do professionals have a duty to minimise cost?*
- *How could staff and patient travel be reduced in our service?*
- *How could we use less energy in heating and lighting in existing buildings, and how can we reduce future energy consumption in any plans for development of the healthcare estate?*
- *What scope do we have in our services for adopting the four principles of sustainable clinical practice?*

- 原则上避免耗尽以经济发展为中心国家的助产士的劳动力。

- 制订一项计划，让助产士访问当地的中小学，并鼓励周围社区的女孩将助产士视为一种职业前景。

财政

假设您是一名临床主任，面临削减预算。一种方法是通过外包清洁和秘书服务来降低后勤服务成本。这虽能减少经济成本，但在医疗卫生保健服务中，却是以牺牲那些薪资最低者的收入为代价（因为没有雇用本单位中最低收入的人）。另一种方法是与周围社区建立更牢固的联系，鼓励招募当地人，这些人更愿意在当地服务，兢兢业业地履行职责而不论其工资水平。

可以将本地采购（而不是外包）应用于运行医疗卫生保健服务的其他方面。临床医生可以考虑多从当地农产品商店采购食物（通常是指在该设施方圆 50 公里范围内种植或采购的食品）。除了通过减少"食物里程"来减少碳排放获得环境效益外，本地采购食物也有助于保留当地经济实力，并在所服务的人群中创造财富。

实现可持续发展需要长期规划，不仅要考虑到与医疗卫生保健设施有关的具体问题，还要考虑到可能影响健康的决定因素。尽管解决医疗服务对健康决定因素的影响所需的范围要比许多医疗卫生保健管理者目前所需要的范围大得多，但现在已经认识到这种方法是必要的。

关于有效系统的进一步思考，请参阅医疗改革系列丛书中第一本的《创建体系》。

■ 思考题

- 向公众会议的成员阐述医疗卫生保健服务预算价值的最佳方式是什么？

- 在寻求更大的价值时，重点应放在边际效应分析上还是放在项目的主要预算上？

- 如何才能最好地鼓励临床医生减少成本投入？

- 采取哪些步骤可以减少不恰当和无效的医疗卫生保健？

- 专业人士是否有责任将成本降至最低？

- 在我们的服务中，如何减少员工和患者的奔波？

- 我们如何减少现有建筑物的供暖和照明中能源的使用，以及如何在医疗产业的所有开发计划中减少未来的能源消耗？

- 采用可持续临床实践四项原则的医疗卫生服务涉及哪些方面？

References

Maximising value and improving outcomes

(1) Kahan JP et al. Measuring the necessity of medical procedures. Medical Care. 1994; 32: 352–365.

(2) Donabedian A. Definition of Quality and Approaches to its Assessment (Explorations in Quality Assessment and Monitoring, Vol 1). Baltimore: Health Administration Press; 1980.

(3) Donabedian A. An Introduction to Quality Assurance in Health Care. Oxford: Oxford University Press; 2002.

(4) Wennberg JE. Tracking Medicine. Oxford: Oxford University Press; 2010.

Seven steps to increase value

(5) Department of Health. England level data by programme budget [data file]. GOV.UK Website https://www.gov.uk/government/publications/2003-04-to-2010-11- programme-budgeting-data. Published August 27, 2012. Accessed August 14, 2014.

(6) Simon HA. Administrative behaviour: a study of decision-making processes in administrative organization. New York: Free Press; 1957. Cited in: Sterman JD. Systems thinking and modeling for a complex world. New York: McGraw-Hill; 2000: 598.

(7) Simon HA. Administrative Behaviour. A study of decision-making processes in administrative organizations. 4th Edition. New York: The Free Press; 1997: 60.

(8) The Health Foundation. STAR: Combining value for money with patient involvement. The Health Foundation Website http://www.health.org.uk/news-and-events/newsletter/star-combining-value-for-money-with-patient-involvement. Updated January 2014. Accessed August 14, 2014.

(9) Gawande A. Complications: A Surgeon's Notes on an Imperfect Science. London: Profile Books Ltd; 2003.

(10) Eddy DM. Three battles to watch in the 1990s. Journal of the American Medical Association. 1993; 270: 520–526.

Responsibility for reducing waste and increasing sustainability

(11) Ohno T. The Toyota Production System. New York: Productivity Press; 1995.

(12) Black J, Miller D. The Toyota Way to Healthcare Excellence: Increase Efficiency and Improve Quality with Lean. Chicago: Health Administration Press; 2008: 236.

(13) Toussaint J, Gerard R, Womack J. On the mend: revolutionizing healthcare to save lives and transform the industry. Cambridge: Lean Enterprise Institute; 2010.

(14) Berwick DM, Hackbarth AD. Eliminating waste in US health care. Journal of the American Medical Association. 2012; 307: 1513–1516.

(15) Department of Health. Annual Report 2005: The Chief Medical Officer on the state of public health. London: The Department; 2006: 17.

参考文献

(16) Nelson EC, Batalden PB, Huber TP, Johnson JK, Godfrey MM, Headrick LA, Wasson JH. Success characteristics of high-performing microsystems: learning from the best. In: Nelson EC, Batalden PB, Godfrey MM (Eds.). Quality by design: a clinical microsystems approach. San Francisco: Jossey-Bass; 2007: 7.

(17) Sibley JC et al. A randomized trial of continuing medical education. New England Journal of Medicine. 1982; 306: 511–515.

(18) Chalmers I, Glasziou P. Avoidable waste in the production and reporting of research evidence. Lancet. 2009; 374: 86–89.

(19) Gallacher K, Montori VM, Mair FS. Understanding Patients' Experiences of Treatment Burden in Chronic Heart Failure Using Normalization Process Theory. Annals of Family Medicine. 2011; 9: 235–243.

(20) Brazier J, Ratcliffe J, Salomon JA, Tsuchiya A. Measuring and Valuing Health Benefits for Economic Evaluation. Oxford: Oxford University Press; 2007: 9.

(21) Maslach C, Leither MP. The Truth About Burnout. San Francisco: Jossey-Bass; 1997. Cited in: Cole TR, Carlin N. The art of medicine: the suffering of physicians. Lancet. 2009; 374: 1414–1415.

(22) Brybye LN, Shanafelt TD. (2011) Physician burnout: a Potential Threat to Successful Healthcare Reform. JAMA. 2011; 305: 2009- 2010.

(23) Saving Carbon, Improving Health. NHS Carbon Reduction Strategy for England. NHS Sustainable Development Unit Website. http://www.sduhealth.org.uk/documents/publications/1237308334_q 2.pdf. Accessed 15 August 2014.

(24) Connor A et al. The carbon footprint of a renal service in the United Kingdom. QJM. 2010; 103: 965–975.

(25) Middleton J. Environmental Health, Climate, Chaos, and Resilience. Medicine, Conflict and Survival. Sandwell's Other Health Summit; 2008: 24: Supplement 1: S63.

(26) Griffiths J, Stewart L. Sustaining a healthy future: taking action on climate change. The Faculty of Public Health; 2008: 12.

(27) Lancet and University College London Institute for Global Health Commission. Managing the health effects of climate change. Lancet. 2009; 373: 1719.

(28) Saving Carbon, Improving Health: UPDATE NHS Carbon Reduction Strategy. NHS Sustainable Development Website. http://www.sduhealth.org.uk/documents/publications/1264693931_k_nhs_carbon_reduction_strategy.pdf. Updated 2010. Accessed July 2014.

(29) Department of Health. Equity and Excellence: Liberating the NHS. 2009.

(30) Mortimer F. The Sustainable Physician. Clinical Medicine. 2010; 10: 110–111.

Part 2
Building blocks for population medicine

The delivery of excellent and equitable population medicine requires three fundamental building blocks – systems of care, networks of people to deliver them, and a supporting culture.

This part comprises four sections

- 2.1 Designing population-based integrated systems
- 2.2 Creating networks to deliver integrated systems of care
- 2.3 Sculpting culture that serves populations

第 2 章
群医学的基本要素

实现卓越而公平的群医学包括三个基本部分：医疗卫生保健体系，开展群医学的人员网络和支持性文化。

本章包括三个部分

- 第 1 节　设计以人群为基础的整合型体系
- 第 2 节　建设可以提供整合型医疗服务的
　　　　　工作网络
- 第 3 节　塑造为群体服务的文化

2.1 Designing population-based integrated systems

As systems are the subject of the first book in our Healthcare Transformation series, we offer only a brief introduction here and encourage you to read Creating Systems.

Having discussed in an earlier section the shift from institutions to systems of care (see section 1.2), we can now explore the definition and design of such systems in relation to population medicine.

■ The definition and design of a system

In the context of population medicine, a system is a set of activities with a common aim and set of objectives, which produces an annual report for the population served, using criteria and standards common to all systems with the same focus.

As the design and development of systems of care is described in Creating Systems, our focus here is to outline the several stages of the design of a system (see Box 2.1), pausing to consider matters of particular relevance to population medicine.

Box 2.1 Stages in the design of a system of care

- Define the scope of the system
- Define the population for which the system has responsibility
- Reach agreement on the aim and objectives for the system
- For each objective, select one or more criteria with which to measure progress
- For each objective, set standards to enable benchmarking and comparison among services
- Reach agreement on the network of organisations necessary to deliver and govern the system (see section 2.2)
- Identify the resources necessary to create a budget for the system (see section 3.4)

The team responsible for system development should have representation from all the key organisations. Consultation should include other people who will be important in making sure the design is implemented. All the organisations and people involved in implementation comprise the 'network'.

第 1 节　设计以人群为基础的整合型体系

　　体系是我们"医疗卫生的转变"系列丛书中第一本书的主题，我们在此仅对其进行简单介绍，鼓励读者自行阅读《创建体系》一书相关章节。

前面章节中已经讨论了医疗卫生保健的提供从机构向体系的转变（详见第 1 章第 2 节），我们现在可以探讨如何定义并设计有关群医学的各种体系了。

■ 体系的定义和设计

　　在群医学的语境下，一个体系是由具有同一目的的一组活动和一系列目标所组成。它们运用那些对一切体系都通用的共同规范和标准，围绕着共同的核心内容，向所服务人群提供年度报告。

　　正如《创建体系》所描述的，设计并开发医疗卫生服务体系的重点在于列出设计体系所需的几个步骤时（专栏 2.1），驻足考虑与群医学特别相关的事项。

专栏 2.1　设计医疗卫生服务体系的步骤

- 界定体系范围；
- 界定体系应该负责的人群；
- 就体系的目的和指标达成共识；
- 就每项具体目标，选择一个或多个指标（criteria）以测量其进展；
- 就每项指标设定标准（standard），以确保各项服务内容可通过基准进行比较；
- 在实施和管理体系时，应就各种机构的网络架构达成共识（见第 2 章第 2 节）；
- 确定该体系所需资源的预算（见第 3 章第 4 节）。

　　负责开发体系的团队应该包括所有关键机构的代表。要与其他重要人员进行磋商确保所设计的体系得以实施，由实施涉及的所有组织和人员组成"工作网络"。

Defining the scope of the system

To define the scope of a system, it is essential to identify the set of activities that need to be coordinated through the system. The scope should be as wide as is necessary to include every activity relevant to the aim. The team leading the development of the system are responsible for facilitating agreement on the activities to be included in the scope. Clarifying terms and definitions from the beginning can save much confusion and can often be a good way to start collaborative engagement: terms such as 'frail elderly' are used frequently without ever being clarified and agreed.

It is usually better to start the discussion about the scope by defining a subgroup of the population, such as 'people at the end of life', rather than a service such as 'palliative care'. Using this approach, the real issue can be identified. For example, a discussion that was intended to develop an urgent care system quickly evolved into a focus on people with multiple morbidities, including both the elderly (the 'frail elderly'), and people under 65 years who have considerable mental health and substance abuse problems. In these cases, developing a Venn diagram is sometimes more useful than compiling a list (Figure 2.1).

Having defined the scope of the system, the next step is to define the population to be served.

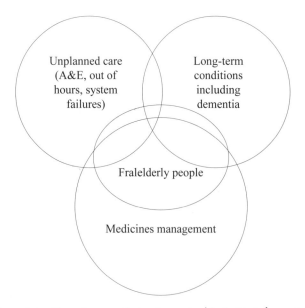

Figure 2.1　The subgroups that make up the 'frail elderly' population

界定体系范围

为了界定体系的范围，必需明确需要通过该体系进行协调的一系列活动。该范围应该尽量广泛，把所有与目标相关的必要活动都纳入其中。领导体系开发的团队负责协调各方，对需纳入服务范围的一系列活动达成共识。

从一开始就澄清术语和定义可以避免引发困惑，通常也是开始协作的好方法：有些术语如"年老体弱者"被频繁地使用，但其含义却从未被界定清楚或取得共识。

通常情况下，从界定一个对象群体的亚人群（"处在生命末期的人群"）入手以开启讨论，其效果更好。而不是以"舒缓医疗"之类的服务内容为入手，来开始相关的讨论。使用这种方法能确定真正的问题所在。例如，旨在发展紧急医疗卫生照护体系的讨论可以迅速演变成针对患有多种疾病人群的讨论，涉及老年人群（"年老体弱者"）和 65 岁以下有严重精神健康问题和药物滥用问题的群体。在这些案例中，制作一张维恩图有时比列表更有用（图 2.1）。

界定了该体系的范围，下一步就要界定所服务的人群。

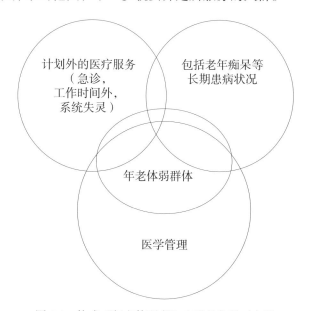

图 2.1　构成"年老体弱者"人群的各种亚人群

Defining the population to be served

Each system of care has responsibility for a defined population. At this stage, it is important to clarify who should constitute the defined population, and to decide upon the optimum size of the population to be served by the system.

In the traditional model of institution-based care, the size of the population served is about 300,000 people, based on the catchment population for a general hospital. The optimum population size for a system of care, however, is a function of inter-related variables as follows.

1. The incidence and prevalence of the problem – the size of the population must be large enough to include the number of clinical events sufficient to enable clinical expertise to be developed and for the production of a meaningful annual report

2. The level of population need for super-specialist services and technology, such as neurosurgery

The implications of these two variables for optimum population size in relation to several different systems of care are shown in Table 2.1.

Table 2.1 The optimum size of population for a system

System focus	Incidence and prevalence	Population need for super-specialist intervention	Optimum population size
Asthma	High	Low	200,000–500,000
Epilepsy	High	High	There may need to be both a local support service for a smaller population – 300,000 –and a neurosurgical service related to a larger population –1 or 2 million – so that the local service's referral rates can be compared.
Parkinson's disease	High	Low	300,000–500,000, although the need for deep brain stimulation may require a larger population size.
Frail elderly people	High	Low	200,000–500,000
Motor neurone disease	Low	High	Support for this uncommon condition requires specialist teams.

Reaching agreement on the aim and objectives

Every system of care should have a single high-level aim with which all professionals and patients can identify. Examples of high-level aims are shown in Display 2.1.

界定所服务人群

每个医疗服务体系都要对某一确定的人群承担职责。在本阶段中，重要的是要确定这一人群是由哪些人所组成，并确定该体系能够服务人群的最佳规模。

在以医疗卫生机构为基础的传统医疗服务模式中，被服务人群的规模约为三十万（300 000），这是基于一个综合医院所能覆盖的地理人群而言。然而，一个医疗服务体系的最佳服务人群规模是取决于以下相互关联的变量：

1. 某种健康问题的发病率和患病率——人群规模必需大到临床事件的数量足以发展临床专业技术并形成有意义的年度报告。

2. 该人群规模应达到需要亚专科（super-specialist）——如神经外科——施展技术和服务的水平。

这两个变量可用于确定几个不同医疗服务体系的最佳人群规模，详见表 2.1。

表 2.1　每个体系中的最佳人群规模

体系的关注内容	发病率和患病率	人群对亚专科干预的需求	最佳人群规模
哮喘	高	低	20 万～50 万人（200 000～500 000）
癫痫	高	高	可能需要同时能针对较小人群的地方性支持服务（30 万人）和对相对较大人群的神经外科服务（100 万或 200 万人），这样就能对各个地方性服务的转诊率进行比较
帕金森病	高	低	30 万～50 万，尽管行脑深部刺激治疗可能需要更大的人群规模
年老体弱者	高	低	20 万～50 万人
运动神经元病	低	高	需要有专家团队对这种罕见病提供技术支持

就目的和具体目标〔aim and objectives〕达成共识

每个医疗服务体系都应有能被所有医疗专业人员和患者识别的、高水准的单一目的。场景 2.1 展示了高水准单一目的的一些例子。

Display 2.1 Examples of organisational aims

Organisation	Aim
NASA	To put a man on the moon and bring him safely back (12 words)
NHS National Breast Cancer Screening Programme	To offer women the opportunity of reducing their risk of dying from breast cancer (14 words)
A hospital	To offer high-quality, safe care tailored to meet the needs of each individual (13 words)

The aim of a system, however, has to be complemented by a set of more detailed objectives on which all those involved in providing care can focus their activities.

A set of objectives suggested for a system for liver disease is presented in Box 2.2.

Box 2.2 Set of objectives suggested for a Liver Disease Programme

- To diagnose and treat liver disease quickly and accurately
- To treat liver disease effectively and safely
- To engage people with the condition and their carers as equal partners
- To promote the health of people with liver disease
- To develop the professionals who support people with liver disease
- To make the best use of resources
- To promote and support research
- To produce an annual report for the population served

There are two main types of objectives for a system of care:
- *clinical objectives, which are analogues of traditional clinical activity, such as 'To diagnose accurately and quickly'*
- *population objectives, relating to the use of resources for the whole population; population objectives are often overlooked by clinicians when setting the objectives for a system*

During the process of objective-setting, the scope may need to be changed. For example, when the set of objectives suggested for liver disease were discussed in a workshop run by public health professionals, an objective to prevent liver disease was introduced:

'To prevent alcoholic liver disease, principally by changing culture and the environment'.

场景 2.1 机构目的范例

机构	目的
美国国家航空航天局	把一人送到月球并安全载回（12 个英文单词）
国家医疗服务体系（NHS）一国家乳腺癌筛查项目	降低妇女的乳腺癌死亡风险（14 个英文单词）
一家医院	为每位患者提供"量身定制"、能满足其需要的、高质量的、安全的医疗服务（13 个英文单词）

然而，该体系的目的仍需由一组更为详细的具体目标补充完善，各项医疗服务也可聚焦这些目标来安排各种活动。专栏 2.2 呈现了一套肝病医疗服务体系的建议目标。

专栏 2.2 针对肝病医疗服务体系的建议目标

- 快速、准确地诊断和治疗肝病。
- 有效、安全地治疗肝病。
- 在患者及其医疗卫生人员之间建立平等的伙伴关系。
- 改善肝病患者群体的健康状况。
- 培训专业人员对肝病患者提供支持。
- 善用各种资源。
- 促进并支持研究工作。
- 向所服务的群体提供年度报告。

医疗服务系统的主要目标有以下两类：

- 临床指标，类似于传统临床活动的指标，如"准确快速地进行诊断"；
- 人群目标，涉及整个人群的资源利用情况；临床医生在为一个体系制定指标时会经常忽视此群体指标。

在设定指标的过程中，其范围可能需要调整。例如，在由公共卫生专业人员主持召开的研讨会上，在讨论针对肝病的系列指标时，会提出预防肝病的指标："主要通过改变文化和环境来预防酒精性肝病"。

■ Questions for reflection

- *What are the main obstacles to the introduction and development of systems in healthcare?*
- *Identify five services including one that is diagnostic in which you are involved or which you know about, e.g. a service for women with pelvic pain. Give each of these services a score on a scale from 1 to 10, where 1 is chaos and 10 represents a perfect system*
- *List three things that institutions are good at doing in healthcare and three things that they fail to do*

■ 思考题

- 在引进和发展医疗卫生保健体系的过程中主要有哪些障碍?

- 确定五项医疗卫生服务,其中包括一项你本人所涉及或了解的诊断,如针对女性盆腔痛的医疗服务。给每项服务打分,评分范围从 1 到 10,"1"代表混乱无序,"10"则代表该医疗服务体系完美无缺。

- 列出各医疗卫生机构在医疗服务领域中三件做得好的服务和三件没做好的服务。

2.2 Creating networks to deliver integrated systems of care

Once a system of care has been designed, the next step is to deliver it to the population in need.

■ The need to shift the focus from structure to systems and networks

In seeking to change the organisation of healthcare, priority has previously been given to changing the structure by:

- *re-organising the bureaucracy*
- *introducing a market*
- *both re-organisation and the introduction of a market*

In population medicine, priority should be given to the development of population-based and integrated systems of care rather than to structural change. Indeed, there is a growing consensus that a new form of organisation is needed to deliver a system of care.

This new form is known as a network. Networks will become the dominant type of organisation in the 21st century, displacing, but not rendering redundant, the bureaucracy, which was the dominant type of organisation in the 20th century.

Although bureaucracies are necessary, they can develop in ways that are unhelpful if they have misguided leadership. One manifestation of over-bureaucratisation is an emphasis on hierarchy, in which senior managers operate in what is known as 'command and control' mode.

Markets have been introduced to varying degrees in the organisation of health services in many countries. In the USA, the role of the market is extensive, whereas in Canada the market's role is much less. In the last 50 years, both bureaucracies and markets have come to dominate the delivery of healthcare.

■ The network, a new type of organisation for healthcare

A new type of organisation for the delivery of healthcare is evolving, known as a network:

> *Networking is a broad concept referring to a form of organized transacting that offers an alternative to either markets or hierarchies. It refers to transactions across an organization's boundaries that are*

第 2 节 建设可以提供整合型医疗服务的工作网络

一旦医疗卫生服务体系设计完成，下一步就是将其应用于需要的人群。

■ 将注意力从结构转向体系和工作网络的需求

在医疗卫生服务的组织机构寻求变革时，以往优先通过以下几个方面对结构进行改变：

- 重组官僚管理体系；
- 引入市场机制；
- 以上两种方式并用。

在群医学中，相对于改变医疗卫生服务体系的结构，应该优先发展基于人群的整合型医疗卫生服务体系。事实上，医疗卫生保健体系需要建立新的组织形式，这一点已得到业内越来越多的共识。

这种新形式即工作网络。工作网络将成为是 21 世纪医疗卫生保健体系的主要形式，取代 20 世纪以官僚体系为主的管理体制，且不会再增加一些冗余工作。

虽然有时官僚体系是必要的，但是如果他们的领导误入歧途，其发展方式是无益的。过度官僚化的一个表现就是强调等级制度，上级管理者只会使用"命令和控制"的方式来推进工作。

在许多国家，市场模式都不同程度地被引入了卫生服务体系。在美国，市场的作用十分强大；而在加拿大，市场的作用则小得多。在过去 50 年中，官僚体制和市场机制已经主导了医疗卫生服务体系的运行。

■ 工作网络，一种医疗卫生保健体系的新型组织形式

一种新型的医疗卫生保健的组织形式正在发展壮大，即工作网络：

工作网络从广义上讲，是指一种有组织的业务来往方式，为市场机制或等级制度提供了替代方案。工作网络是超越某个机构（专业、职能）范围之外与其他一些合作伙伴的经常、持续交往。这种

recurrent and involve continuing relationships with a set of partners. The transactions are coordinated and controlled on a mutually agreed basis that is likely to require common protocols and systems, but do not necessarily require direct supervision by the organization's own staff. (1)

Networks as organisations are different from hierarchies. As emphasised by Wright, networks are not 'top down'.

A network ... emerges from the bottom up; individuals function as autonomous nodes, negotiating their own relationships, forging ties, coalescing into clusters. There is no 'top' in a network; each node is equal and self-directed. Democracy is a kind of network; so is a flock of birds, or the World Wide Web. (2)

Wright's definition of a network introduces the term 'node', which also helps to differentiate networks from hub-and-spoke organisations. A hub-and-spoke organisation implies that one partner is more important than the others, whereas in a network all the partners – the professor, the generalist, and the patient – are all 'nodes' of equal importance but have different roles.

Networks and teams

Within a bureaucracy, teams play a very important part in delivering care. The importance of good teamwork, particularly multidisciplinary teamwork, is increasingly being recognised.

There are important differences between teams and networks (see Display 2.2).

Display 2.2 The differences between teams and networks

Teams	Networks
Members all work in the same organisation	Members come from different organisations
Communication is primarily face-to-face	Face-to-face contact is usually infrequent
One member is usually designated as the person who has bureaucratic authority by the organisation in which the team works	It is uncommon for one person to have bureaucratic control

Networks are developed through sapiential authority, that is, an authority based on knowledge.

业务往来基于合作伙伴之间的共识来共同协作管理，有可能需要遵循统一的操作规范和工作流程，但不一定需要组织内部成员直接监督管理[1]。

组织的工作网络和等级管理体系是不同的，如怀特所说，工作网络不是"自上而下"的管理方式。

工作网络是自下而上产生的，个体充当自治节点，协商彼此关系，建立合作组带并集结成群落。在工作网络中没有上级领导，每一个节点都是平等的、自主的。所谓"民主"就是一种"网络"；一群鸟或万维网都是某种形式的工作网络[2]。

怀特在工作网络的定义中引入了"节点"一词，以此区分工作网络和中心辐射式组织。中心辐射式组织意味着其中一个合作伙伴比其他都重要，而工作网络中所有的合作伙伴——包括教授、全科医生和患者这些"节点"——都同样重要，但是发挥不同的作用。

工作网络和团队

在官僚体系中，团队在提供医疗卫生服务方面有着十分重要的作用。团队合作的重要性，特别是多学科团队合作，越来越得到业界的认可。

团队和工作网络有着明显的区别（场景 2.2）。

场景 2.2　团队和工作网络的区别

团　队	工作网络
所有成员都在一个机构工作	成员均来自不同的机构
主要通过面对面交流	面对面交流不是很频繁
通常一个成员被机构指定为负责人来领导团队的工作	一般不会指定一个负责人

工作网络通常是通过智性权威（即基于知识的权威性）发展而来的。

Types of network

Although networks run primarily on trust rather than on hierarchical authority, some of the relationships within a network are governed by formal rules of conduct, or sometimes contracts.

Accountable Care Organisations and new approaches

In several countries, a more formal split has been established between organisations that pay for healthcare, such as insurance companies, and those who provide healthcare. In NHS England, it is the role of the commissioner to pay for healthcare. With the development of this formal split, a type of network is emerging that has a greater degree of bureaucratic, contractual formality than has been the case hitherto. The term for such an organisation in the USA is the Accountable Care Organisation (ACO).

ACOs consist of providers who are jointly held accountable for achieving measured quality improvements and reductions in the rate of spending growth. (3)

The term Accountable Care Organisation has been used in the NHS although it has not been generally adopted. There is recognition, however, of the need to develop networks that have more formality than groups of professionals with a common interest.

One model is for one of the services to be given a contract to act as the 'prime contractor' or 'prime provider', responsible for involving all the other relevant services and, where necessary, issuing a subcontract. This type of organisation:

- *is responsible for ensuring that integrated care is delivered to a defined population within a fixed budget to explicit quality standards and outcomes*
- *will need a lead clinician skilled in population medicine, one of whose responsibilities will be to produce an explicit care pathway or care map which most patients should follow through the network*

Another approach is for those who pay for healthcare to change the type of contract they use. Traditionally, payers contracted with the main islands in the archipelago of healthcare – hospitals, primary care, community services and mental health services (see Figure 1.9). Such contracts were focused on price and volume supported by a few quality indicators, such as waiting list times. A new approach uses population- and outcomes-based incentivised contracts so that all

工作网络的类型

尽管工作网络的运作主要靠彼此的信任而非等级关系，网络内机构之间的关系通常也需要受到正式的行为准则或合同管辖。

责任医疗组织（Accountable Care Organisations）和新合作方式

在一些国家，医疗卫生服务的支付机构（如保险公司）和服务机构已经正式分开。在 NHS 中，特定的行政长官负责支付医疗卫生的相关费用。在医疗卫生服务的支付机构和服务机构正式分离的过程中，形成了一种更加繁复、更拘泥于合同形式的工作网络。在美国，这类机构叫作"责任医疗组织"（ACO）。

> 责任医疗组织是由那些对提高医疗卫生保健服务的质量和降低其支出增长率承担共同责任的服务提供者所组成[3]。

责任医疗组织这个名词曾经在英国国家医疗服务体系使用过，不过没有被广泛采纳。然而，业界一致认为建立一种更加正式的工作网络十分必要，而非仅靠一些兴趣相投的专业团队在一起工作。

这种责任医疗组织的一种运作模式是把其中一个机构作为"主合同方"或"主要服务提供方"，与其签订合同，负责统筹其他参与机构的工作，并在必要时与其他机构签订子合同。这类机构：

- 负责保证在一定预算范围内确定的人群得到整合医疗卫生服务，而且这种服务有明确的质量标准和目标效果。

- 需要由精通群医学的临床医生领导，其职责之一是建立清楚明确的医疗卫生服务路径或服务路线，让大部分患者可通过工作网络接受医疗服务。

另外一种运作模式是由医疗卫生保健服务支付者来改变他们的合约模式。传统方式是支付方和众多医疗卫生保健提供方中的主体部分（如医院、初级卫生保健机构、社区服务机构及精神卫生机构，图 1.9）等签订合同。合同内容侧重于价格以及符合一些质量指标（如预约等候时间）的服务数量。新的运作模式是签订基于人群和服务结果的、带有激励机制的合同，激

the relevant clinicians from the different provider organisations are incentivised to work together focused on the needs of all the people with a particular disease in a population.

Variables affecting the development of an effective network for integrated care

When developing a network for integrated care, several variables can influence what it is possible to achieve, including:

- *the management style of the health service*
- *the degree to which the network is related to a system of care with a clear, written plan recognised by the principal organisations involved*
- *the degree of authority given to the person charged with leading or coordinating the network*
- *the support provided to the individual identified as the coordinator (for example, has the coordinator been given protected time and administrative and IT support to arrange meetings, or information- scientist support to create a website and a virtual community?)*

These variables are representative of the influences participating organisations need to discuss.

■ Ending the era of primary and secondary care

For the specialist who has responsibility for a population and is developing a network, it is vital to create a culture in which everyone is considered to be of equal importance. This is not always easy to achieve:

- *medicine has become split into primary and secondary care, which can be counterproductive when building a system*
- *a prejudice remains that some clinicians are of lower status than others*

This prejudice is reinforced when the issue of 'missed diagnosis' in general practice is raised by hospital specialists or the issue of over-use of resources by specialists is raised by general practitioners.

> *'It was an easy diagnosis. How did those guys miss it?' Hospital doctor speaking about general practitioners 'Why do they keep doing all these tests? They've lost their clinical judgment.' General practitioners speaking about hospital doctors*

Although such criticism is sometimes justified, it is usually made by a clinician who is not familiar with the difference between sensitivity and positive predictive value (see Box 2.3). Moreover, this criticism highlights an important consideration in population medicine regarding the different perspectives of clinicians who are providing different types of care for people in the population served:

励所有相关的来自不同医疗卫生保健提供方的临床医生共同努力，来满足人群中的特定疾病患者的服务需求。

影响整合型医疗卫生服务网络有效运行的各种因素

在建立整合型医疗卫生服务网络时，以下几个因素会影响其工作效果：

- 医疗卫生服务的管理模式；
- 工作网络中的主要服务机构制订的清晰书面计划在多大程度上可以将整个网络与医疗卫生服务体系融合一体；
- 工作网络领导者或协调者的权限大小；
- 协调者得到的支持程度（如：是否保障协调者有足够的时间及足够的行政和信息技术支持来组织会议，或是否有信息技术专家的支持以建立网站和虚拟社区）。

以上这些都是影响工作网络效果的代表性因素，需要参与机构仔细讨论。

■ 初级和二级卫生保健时代的结束

对负有人群责任、要建立医疗卫生保健网络的专科医生来说，创立一种每个人都同等重要的文化氛围十分重要。这不是很容易做到，因为：

- 医学已经被分割成初级卫生保健和二级卫生保健，这两部分在建立卫生服务体系时可能是互相抵触的。
- 现在仍存在一种偏见，认为某些临床医生的地位低于其他医生。

当医院专科医生指出全科医疗中出现的漏诊问题，或者全科医生认为医院专科医生过度使用资源时，这种偏见更被强化了。

医院的医生会这样指责全科医生："这种疾病很容易诊断，那些医生怎么能漏诊呢？"。全科医生又会说医院的专科医生："为什么他们总是做这么多化验检查呢？他们连最基本的临床判断都没有吗？"。

尽管类似指责有时也不无道理，但这种指责通常出自不懂灵敏度和阳性预测值区别的临床医生之口（专栏2.3）。此外，这种指责凸显了群医学中的一个重点考虑因素，即为患者人群提供不同类型医疗卫生服务临床医生们的不同视角：

- *the perspective of the clinician in primary care, who is the first point of contact for the general population*
- *the perspective of the clinician in secondary care, who sees only those patients who have been filtered for referral by the clinician who was the first point of contact – these patients represent a subset of the population*

As the prevalence of disease in the general population is different from that in the population subset who have been referred, the positive predictive value for every test is different.

Box 2.3 Definitions of sensitivity and positive predictive value

Sensitivity: the proportion of people with the disease who are identified as having it by a positive test result

Positive predictive value: the probability that a person with a positive test result actually has the disease (4)

Furthermore, the neurosurgeon who says that haemorrhagic stroke is an 'easy' diagnosis because all the patients reaching the service complain of atypical headache in middle age is failing to appreciate that, although almost all of the patients who have had a stroke will report that they had an atypical headache, if every general practitioner referred every patient with atypical headache the specialist service would collapse.

In building a community of practice, it may be more helpful to use the terms generalists and specialists, although the use of this terminology could also have pejorative connotations. Although specialists may know more about a particular specialty, specialists and generalists deal with different subgroups in the population served.

When building a system of care and creating a community of practice to work within that system, it is important to encourage a culture change in which people refer to all the clinicians serving a population, and the terms primary and secondary care are made redundant.

When building a new culture, language is vital.

■ Making care pathways

As the delivery of care becomes more complicated, both patients and clinicians can benefit from care pathways, which describe the path a patient with a particular problem usually follows through the network. The term 'care pathways' or 'integrated care pathways' (ICP), however, is used in different ways. A team in Scotland has identified three different meanings associated with the term integrated care pathway (see Box 2.4). (5)

- 初级卫生保健的临床医生视角：这些医生通常是一般大众最先接触的医务工作者。
- 二级卫生保健医生的视角，他们仅诊治那些经过初级卫生保健医生初步"筛选"转诊的患者，这些患者代表了人群的一部分。

疾病的患病率在普通人群和被转诊的那部分人群中是不同的，因此每种检测的阳性预测值是不同的。

专栏 2.3　灵敏度和阳性预测值的定义

灵敏度：具有某种疾病的人得到阳性检测结果的比率
阳性预测值：一个有阳性结果的人实际患某种疾病的可能性[4]

此外，神经外科医生认为出血型脑卒中"很容易诊断"，是因为在专科被诊断为脑卒中的中年患者都出现非典型性头痛；这些神经外科医生没有意识到，虽然确诊为脑卒中的所有患者几乎都报告有非典型性头痛，但如果全科医生把每一位有非典型性头痛的患者都转诊给他们，专科医疗服务就会崩溃。

在构建医疗卫生服务共同体时，用全科医生和专科医生这样的名词可能会更有帮助，尽管这两个术语的使用有时略带贬义。专科医生可能在某一特定领域了解得更多，但专科医生和全科医生是为总人群中的不同群体服务的。

在构建医疗卫生保健体系和建立医疗卫生保健共同体时，重要的是要转变人们认为所有医生均服务于同一人群的文化误区。初级卫生保健和二级卫生保健这类术语实则多余。

当构建一个新的文化的时候，语言是十分重要的。

■ 建立医疗卫生保健的服务路径

由于提供医疗卫生保健服务的模式越来越复杂，患者和医生都可以从照护路径上获益。照护路径即一个有特定疾病的患者在医疗卫生保健的工作网络内通常要遵循的路径。然而，"医疗卫生保健路径"和"整合型医疗卫生保健路径（ICP）"两个名词的使用方法不同。一个苏格兰团队提出了"整合型医疗卫生保健路径"这一术语的三个不同含义（专栏 2.4）[5]。

Box 2.4 Different meanings attributed to the term 'integrated care pathway' (5)

1. The actual care process experienced by each individual patient: in the literature, this is represented as a journey in which the patient is the traveller

2. Maps that define best practice and the minimum clinical standards or essential components of care for every patient in a given situation: a care pathway is a standard or universal plan for how a patient with a particular condition will be treated

3. Physical documentation located at each point of care, central to the task of care as the patient travels the pathway. The care process, the place on that pathway, and anticipated future progress, are all clearly presented on the documentation for all those involved to see

Resistance to the development of care pathways

There has been professional resistance to the development of care pathways which some clinicians claim will lead to standardisation or 'cookbook' medicine. Although such criticisms need to be addressed, one powerful way to tackle widespread unwarranted variation in clinical practice is through the use of care pathways. In addition, standardisation of certain aspects of clinical care enables the inexperienced clinician to concentrate on an individual patient's anxieties and concerns and to personalise the patient's care, rather than trying to remember which post-operative fluid regime a particular surgeon prefers. Therefore, standardisation is particularly important when care is delivered by inexperienced clinicians.

The way in which pathways are introduced can reduce the level of resistance. For example, it is important to emphasise that some items in the pathway need to be localised or can be changed because of local circumstances, such as the names and contact details of key local services or the opportunity to offer a patient entry into a randomised controlled trial, whereas some items should not be varied, such as the prescription of a drug that is supported by very strong evidence and national guidance.

■ The inevitability of networking

Manuel Castells, one of the intellectual giants of the last 50 years, describes how networks are driving what he calls the Third Industrial Revolution (6). Castells cites the three drivers of this revolution as citizens, knowledge, and the Internet. Following technological developments over the last five years, it is now possible to substitute the smartphone for the Internet. Although Castells' analysis does not include healthcare,

专栏 2.4 整合医疗卫生保健路径的不同含义 (5)

1. 每个患者实际所经历的医疗卫生保健照护过程：这在文献中可以被描述为一次旅程，而每个患者就是一个旅行者。

2. 路径图就是每个患者在特定情况下可得到的最佳医疗卫生保健照护以及该照护的最低临床标准或必要组成内容：单个照护路径是有特定疾病患者所接受治疗的规范化或通用型方案。

3. 患者接受医疗照护过程中，在每个照护节点都有记录首要任务的实物文档。过程、路径中的各个节点以及预期的进展都会清晰地记录在文档中，以供所有相关人员人参考。

建立医疗卫生照护路径的阻碍

在建立医疗卫生照护路径时，存在一些来自专业人员的阻力，一些临床医生认为这会导致标准化医疗或"按图索骥式"医疗。尽管批评提出的问题要予以解决，但要解决临床工作中普遍存在的不合理问题，一种有效的方法就是使用医疗照护路径。此外，临床照护中某些方面采取标准化操作可使那些经验不足的临床医生能更专注于处理患者个体的焦虑和担忧的情绪，为患者提供个性化的服务，而不必费心记住一些无关紧要之事，如某个外科医生更喜欢用哪种术后输液方案。因此，标准化对于经验不足的临床医生提供医疗卫生照护时尤为重要。

医疗卫生照护路径的引入方式可以降低某些阻力。例如，在引入路径时应强调：根据当地的具体情况，路径的一些内容尚待"本土化"或需根据本地情况修正，如当地主要照护机构的名称及联系方式或患者纳入随机对照试验的机会等；而有些内容是不能改变的，比如某种有充分证据和国家指南支持的药品处方。

■ 建立医疗卫生工作网络的必然性

曼纽尔·卡斯特是过去半个世纪间的科学巨人之一，他描述网络是如何驱动被他称之为"第三次工业革命"兴起的 (6)。卡斯特认为：公民、知识和互联网是这次革命的三项驱动因素。基于过去 5 年来的科技发展，用智能手机代替互联网现已成为可能。尽管卡斯特的分析不包括医疗卫生，但同

it is highly relevant to the development of health services in the 21st century. In this context, the driving forces in organisational development are patients, knowledge and the Internet, all of which interact with one another.

The Internet, by its very nature, promotes networks. It is not merely a passive transmitter of bits of information; it facilitates the creation of knowledge, for example, within healthcare, by allowing instant feedback from patients. The Internet helps to create what has been called a networked information economy.

The network will be the dominant type of organisation in the 21st century. In part this is due to the Internet, but it is also due to the recognition that the bureaucracy and the market, dominant types of organisation of the 20th century, have severe limitations.

■ The network as a complex adaptive system

Networks offer a response to the complexity that is healthcare with both a personalised and a population view to be considered. The resultant networks have been referred to as complex adaptive systems: flexible, resilient and evolving.

To function as a complex adaptive system, a health service network requires the different types of clinician, who are clear about their respective roles within the network and their responsibilities towards the population served, to work together to increase value for the whole population in need.

■ Questions for reflection

- *Think of the best clinical network you know and list at least three of the network's characteristics that might explain its success*
- *Think of a clinical network you know that does not work well and list at least three of the network's characteristics that might explain its poor performance*
- *Imagine you are the chief executive of a hospital: what would be your main concerns about the involvement of 'your' clinicians in clinical networks?*

References

(1) Child J. Organization. Contemporary Principles and Practice. New Jersey: Blackwell Publishing; 2005: 15.

(2) Wright A. Glut: Mastering information through the ages. Washington DC: Joseph Henry Press; 2005: 7.

(3) McLellan M, McKethan AN, Lewis JL, Roski J, Fisher ES. A National Strategy to put

21 世纪的医疗卫生服务发展密切相关。在这一背景下，医疗服务机构发展的驱动力就是患者、知识和互联网，它们彼此相互影响。

互联网本身的特性也会推动工作网络的发展。它不仅是信息的被动传播载体，还有推进知识创造过程的功能：比如在医疗服务中，可以通过互联网得到患者的即时反馈信息。互联网有助于创造所谓的网络信息经济。

工作网络将成为 21 世纪组织的主要运作形式。这在一定程度上要归功于互联网的发展，同时也与人们意识到官僚机构和市场这两种 20 世纪占主导地位的组织形式有着的严重局限性有关。

■ 工作网络是一个复杂适应系统

医疗卫生工作网络要应对以下两个复杂方面：既要考虑个人想法，又要兼顾人群视角。由此产生的工作网络被称为复杂适应系统，其特点是：灵活、适应力强且可不断调整完善。

要让这个复杂适应系统发挥功效，提供医疗服务的工作网络需要有不同类型的临床医生的共同参与。这些临床医生要明确自己在工作网络中的角色和对所服务人群的责任，才能共同为整个需要帮助的人群创造价值。

■ 思考题

• 思考一下你所知的最好的临床工作网络，并列举至少 3 个令其成功的特点。

• 思考一下你所知的效果不佳的临床工作网络，并列举至少 3 个令其表现不佳的特征。

• 如果你是一个医院的首席执行官：在让手下临床医生融入到临床工作网络方面，你最关注的问题是什么？

参考文献

Accountable Care Into Practice. Health Affairs. 2010; 29(5): 982.

(4) Gray JAM. Evidence-Based Healthcare. London: Churchill Livingstone; 2009.

(5) NHS Scotland. A Workbook for People Starting to Develop Integrated Care Pathways. 2009.

(6) Castells M. The Network Society. Cheltenham: Edward Elgar; 2004.

2.3 Sculpting culture that serves populations

As culture is the subject of Book 3 in our Healthcare Transformation series, we offer only a brief introduction here and encourage you to read Creating Culture.

■ The influence of culture

Culture is one of the key components of a health service (Figure 2.2), although the paramount importance of culture in a healthcare setting has been recognised only in the last 10 years. In previous decades, those who manage healthcare were preoccupied with structure and financial regulation and, more recently, quality and safety systems. There is now a need to focus explicitly on the culture of a healthcare organisation.

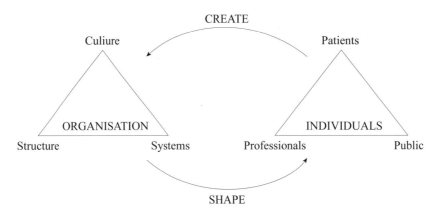

Figure 2.2　The key components of a health service

It is important to acknowledge that culture influences not only decision-making in an organisation, but also the way in which people behave.

... assumptions, values and patterns of behaviour within an organization are often termed its 'organizational culture'. (1)

It is also important to be aware of and recognise the presence of any subcultures within the culture of a health service. The existence of subcultures is determined by three principal influences.

第 3 节　塑造为群体服务的文化

因为文化是我们"卫生转型系列丛书"第三册的主题，因此，我们在此仅简要介绍，并鼓励你阅读《创建文化》一书。

■ 文化的影响

文化是医疗卫生服务的关键组成部分之一（图 2.2），尽管人们在过去10 年间才认识到文化是一个医疗卫生机构的命脉。在过去的几十年间，那些医疗服务的管理者们一直全神贯注于卫生体系的结构和财政监管，近些年又开始关注该体系的质量和安全问题。现在，确有必要聚焦于阐明一个医疗服务机构的文化内涵。

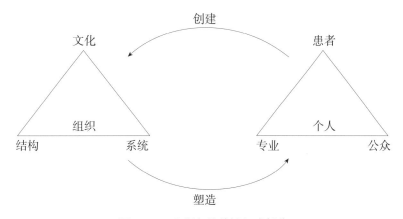

图 2.2　卫生服务的关键组成部分

重要的是，我们必须承认，文化不仅影响一个组织机构的决策，而且也影响人们的行为方式。

……组织内的设想、价值观和行为模式通常被称为其"组织文化"[1]。

还有重要的一点是，要意识并认识到在医疗卫生服务的文化内存在着各种亚文化。这些亚文化的存在受到了以下三个主要因素的影响：

1. The power of national or international cultures relating to a particular specialty: in every country, the culture of a cardiothoracic service is different from that of a paediatric service, and both differ from the culture of a mental health service

2.The nature of the prevailing leadership, for instance, the culture of a particular cardiothoracic or paediatric service may differ greatly from that of another within the same health service

3.The development of counter-cultures in opposition to the culture created by the official senior leaders of an organisation. There are two main types of counter-culture: formal and informal. The Board of a hospital may regard the trade union as a counter-culture, but it has a formal standing. An informal counter-culture in a hospital might be one of heavy drinking, or there may a racist subculture

■ Culture needed to promote population health

The culture needed to promote population health is shown in Box 2.5. The culture for population health is not the type of 'command and control' culture that evolves when a single department or institution pursues a particular target. Although it has been popular for the last few decades, there is increasing evidence that the approach of pressing people to perform well and rewarding them financially if they do so is not only less effective than was originally thought but also has severe adverse effects (2, 3). Furthermore, a culture in which institutions compete with one another for prestige, power and money results in behaviour by which other services are exploited or even deceived.

Box 2.5 The culture of population healthcare

- All the agencies involved are focused on the population to be served, not their own well-being
- People in one organisation are concerned about possible adverse effects of their decisions on other organisations and seek to mitigate them
- Individuals and individual organisations behave altruistically, that is, they may take decisions or behave in ways that are not advantageous to their particular position in the short term

Sculpting a culture of respect

It is common for clinicians in specialist services to speak with disrespect of clinicians in the generalist service, often without experience of having worked in general practice.

There is a need to move towards a culture in which clinicians in specialist services speak with respect of clinicians in the generalist service because in population medicine all clinicians are of equal standing although they may perform different jobs.

1. 与特定专业相关的国家或国际文化的力量：在每个国家，胸外科的服务文化必然不同于儿科的服务文化，而这两者又都与精神卫生科的服务文化有所差异。

2. 领导层的风格不同。例如，某特定团队的胸外科或儿科的服务文化，可能与在同一系统中的另一个团队差异甚大。

3. 与组织内资深领导者所创立文化相对立的非主流文化的发展。非主流文化主要有两种类型：正式的和非正式的。医院董事会可能把工会视为一种非主流文化，但工会具有正式的地位。在某医院里，非正式的非主流文化之一可能是酗酒，或是存在某种种族主义亚文化。

■ 促进群体健康所需的文化

促进人群健康所需的文化如专栏 2.5 所示。群体健康文化不是由哪个单一部门或机构为追求特定目标而形成的"命令和控制"文化。尽管在过去几十年里，这种文化一直很流行，但越来越多的证据表明，逼迫人们表现出色并给予经济奖励的方法不仅没有原先认为的有效，而且还具有严重的副作用[2, 3]。此外，各机构之间为了威望、权力和金钱而相互竞争的文化环境，可导致其他服务内容被削减甚至发生欺骗行为。

专栏 2.5　人群医疗卫生保健的文化

- 所有相关机构所关注的是其服务的人群而非自身的福祉。
- 在一个组织中，人们所关心的是自己的决策是否会给其他组织带来的不利影响并想方设法减轻这些影响。
- 个人和各个组织的行为是利他的，他们可能做出的决定或行为在短期内对他们特定的地位不利。

塑造相互尊重的文化

一个常见的状况是，从事专科服务的临床医生虽然没有在全科领域的工作经验，却经常会对从事全科医学服务的医生出言不逊。

文化建设应当朝着这么一个方向发展：从事专科的临床医生尊重从事全科的医生，平等对话。因为在群医学中，所有临床医生虽然可能从事的工种不同，但地位一律平等。

Culture and leadership

Culture and leadership are inter-related. Leadership shapes culture, and functions such as management and administration then act within that culture.

(1) This principle is very important to successful organisations like Toyota because:

> *An organization's culture defines what goes on in its workplace. Loosely defined, culture is the soft, imprecise, fuzzy stuff of everyday life. Within any company, it is what people think and believe and what drives daily priorities. (4)*

For the clinician with an interest in population medicine, being a leader and therefore shaping all aspects of culture is part of the job.

The shift in healthcare provision from a paradigm concerned with those patients in contact with a service to one concerned with the population served requires a considerable cultural change. A culture concerned with the population served exhibits the characteristics shown in Box 2.6.

Box 2.6 Characteristics of a healthcare culture concerned with the population served

- In documents describing the service, there are frequent references to the population served, not only reports about the quality of care delivered to the proportion of the population in contact with the service but also about the population in need, the level of unmet need, and degree of variation in referral rates to the hospital service according to referring practice and socio-economic group of patient
- Maps are the artefacts that indicate whether a service is concerned with the population. Although maps are rarely visible in hospitals, the service providing care for a population will have numerous maps on display, which provide a key source of information for a population-based health service: for example, maps showing isochrones of the time taken to travel to the hospital from different housing estates in the locality, subpopulations in which there is a high incidence of disease or from which there is a high referral rate. The identification of variation often reveals cultural differences

This shift in paradigm, however, is one change among several that need to take place if the culture of healthcare organisations is to be transformed from that which was appropriate for the 20th century to that which is appropriate for the 21st century. The various shifts in health service culture that need to take place are summarised in Figure 2.3.

文化和领导力

文化和领导力是有内在关联的。领导层塑造文化并在该文化下行使各种管理和行政职能[1]。此原理对丰田公司这类成功的企业而言非常重要。因为:

> 一个组织的文化界定了其工作场所该如何运营。从广义上讲,文化指的是每天日常生活中那些软性的(soft)、难以精确表达(impresice)和模糊(fuzzy stuff)的内容。在任何一家公司里,文化是人们所想所信以及日常重点工作的驱动力[4]。

对于热衷于群医学的临床医生而言,作为领导者并因此塑造服务文化的方方面面,则是其工作的一部分。

范式从"向'上门求医的患者'提供服务"转化为"向'对所服务人群'提供关注",需要进行重大的文化变革。专栏 2.6 展示了与'所服务人群'有关的文化特征。

专栏 2.6　与所服务人群有关的医疗卫生文化特征

- 在描述医疗卫生保健服务的文件中,经常会引用到"所服务人群"的信息;内容不仅涉及到直接受益人群(如患者,仅占此人群的一部分)所获得的卫生服务的质量,也涉及到那些有需要的人群以及他们尚有哪些未得到满足的医疗卫生保健服务需要,还要报告由于患者所处的不同社会经济群体是否影响到医院的转诊过程和转诊率等方面。
- 从绘制的各类路径图中,可以看出该服务是否真正关注到了应该涉及的人群。尽管在医院里很少能看到此类路径图,但为人群提供的医疗卫生服务中,此类路径图却处处可见且提供了重要的信息。例如,可绘制当地从不同住宅区到医院所花时间的等时线地图,发病率高或转诊率高的亚人群之所在位置。这些差异的识别往往可以揭示出文化的不同。

然而,如果要将医疗卫生机构的文化从 20 世纪转变为 21 世纪,范式的转变仅仅是诸多需要进行的变革之一。图 2.3 总结了卫生服务文化中需要发生的几类变革。

20th Century Care	21sh Century Care
Clinician-centred	Parient-centred
Patient as passive complier	Citizen as co-producer of wellbeing
Focus on cure and effectiveness	Focus on prevention, care & harm
Increase quality	Reduce waste and increase quality
Good care for known patienis	Equitable care for populations
Hospital as focus	Focus on systems
Public sector bureaucracy	Pluralistic networds
Driven by finance	Driven digitally by knowledge
High carbon usage	Low carbon usage
Challenges met by growth	Challanges met by transtormation

Figure 2.3　The transformation in 20th century healthcare culture to meet the needs of the 21st century

■ The influence of leadership

Any leader influences culture through what they say and, importantly, through the way in which they behave. For clinicians leading a service concerned with the population served, it is essential to control:

- *the editorial content of any documents produced*
- *the appearance of buildings relevant to the health service and the environment in which care is provided*

When embarking upon culture change, these aspects of the service convey messages about the organisation's culture, not only to the population served but also to the wider general public.

It is important to be explicit about culture. Ten years ago it would have been rare to discuss the culture of an organisation, whereas now it is common and should be universal. Although the leaders of an organisation must be aware of their behaviour, they also need to think more about the language they use because language is the dominant determinant in the culture of an organisation. It is also the main way in which culture is conveyed to people who come into contact with the organisation or to the people who join it.

Although the concept of an organisation's 'culture' can sometimes seem nebulous, there are discrete explicit steps that can be taken to influence culture by shaping the language used and the concepts that prevail.

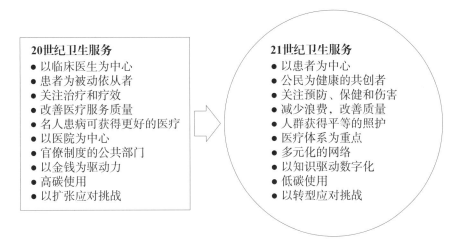

图 2.3　为适应 21 世纪的需求，20 世纪的医疗卫生保健文化需要进行的变革

■ 领导力的影响

任何一名领导者都会通过其言论——更为重要的是通过其行为方式——来影响所在组织机构的文化。对于为人群提供医疗服务的临床医生而言，有必要对以下方面进行管控：

•组织机构编制的任何文件的内容；

•与医疗服务相关的建筑物外观以及提供医疗卫生保健服务的环境情况。

当进行文化变革时，这些服务内容不仅向所服务的人群，也向广大民众传递了与机构文化相关的信息。

精准阐明文化内容十分重要。如果说十年前探讨组织文化还是十分罕见，那么现在这已变得常见，而且还应推广普及。尽管一个组织的领导者们不仅必须意识到其行为对机构文化的影响，他们也需更多地考虑所使用的语言，因为语言是组织文化中的主要决定因素。这也是将文化传达给外部接触者或内部人员的主要方式。

虽然一个组织的"文化"概念有时看起来模糊不清，但仍可采用具体精准的步骤——包括塑造所用语言和各种主流理念——来影响文化。

Although the behaviour of leaders is important in creating a new culture, or in shaping an existing culture, it is necessary to complement behaviour at a senior management level with measures to ensure that all people are cognisant of the culture change and act accordingly.

The role of leadership in population medicine is further explored in section 3.1.

Any new culture needs to be inculcated from the first day of professional education. Some medical schools have already recognised the need for a new curriculum to meet the demands and pressures of a world in which there are finite resources, as outlined by Cooke in the New England Journal of Medicine:

We must ensure that all students acquire a basic understanding of how medical care is financed, where national healthcare policies come from, and the politics that shape financing and workforce choices. (5)

This task of culture change will not be easy. Clinicians must continue to be committed to the individual patients in front of them, but will also need to develop a commitment to the whole population in need, including to those patients they have never seen and may never see.

References

(1) Schein EH. Organizational Culture and Leadership. New Jersey: John Wiley & Sons Inc; 2004.

(2) Seddon J. Freedom from Command and Control. Buckingham: Vanguard Consulting Ltd; 2003.

(3) Gardner HK. Performance Pressure as a Double Edged Sword. Administrative Science

尽管在创造新文化或打造现有文化方面，领导者的行为很重要，但仍有必要在高级管理层的文化方面采取额外措施，以确保所有人都认识到文化的变化并按其行事。

在群医学领域中，有关领导能力的作用将于本书的第 3 章第 1 节进一步阐述。

要想使新文化扎根，就必须让学生在接受专业教育的第一天就沐浴在这种文化氛围中，反复熏陶。一些医学院校已经认识到需要设立一个新课程来应对在资源有限的世界里所面临的需求和压力。正如库克在《新英格兰医学杂志》上总结所言：

> 我们必须确保所有学生对医疗卫生保健的筹资方式、国家医疗政策的起源以及决定筹资和人力资源选择的方针政策有一个基本的了解[5]。

实现文化变革的目标绝非易事。临床医生必须致力于服务于其面对的每位患者，同时也需要对所有需要帮助的人群做出承诺，包括那些他们尚未谋面和可能永远素昧平生的患者。

───────── 参 考 文 献 ─

Quarterly. 2012; 57: 1–46.

(4) Morgan JM, Liker JK. The Toyota Product Development System: Integrating people, process, and technology. New York: Productivity Press; 2006: 217-218.

(5) Cooke M. Cost consciousness in Patient Care – What is Medical Education's responsibilities? New England Journal of Medicine. 2010; 362: 1253–1254.

Part 3

Developing skills for population medicine

This part comprises four sections

- 3.1 Leadership that serves populations
- 3.2 Quality improvement that serves populations
- 3.3 Managing knowledge that serves populations
- 3.4 Creating budgets for populations

第 3 章
发展群医学技能

本章包括四个部分

- 第 1 节　为人群服务的领导力
- 第 2 节　为提升人群服务的质量
- 第 3 节　为各种人群服务的知识管理
- 第 4 节　为人群制订预算

3.1 Leadership that serves populations

In this section, we address six key questions regarding leadership in population medicine:

- *What do we mean by leadership?*
- *What is the purpose of leadership in population medicine?*
- *What is different about leadership in population medicine?*
- *What are the key leadership requirements in population medicine?*
- *How do we measure leadership performance in population medicine?*
- *What are the roles and priorities of current leaders?*

■ What do we mean by leadership?

> *There are almost as many different definitions of leadership as there are persons who have attempted to define the concept. (1)*

An important distinction between the functions of leadership and management was provided in section 2.3. A further challenge lies in the distinction between the various uses and understandings of the term leadership itself. The challenge associated with agreeing a single definition of leadership is well known. A different question is, 'What do we mean by leadership?'

A common point of confusion lies with the (often interchangeable) use of the terms leader and leadership. In this book, the term leadership is used to describe a set of values-based behaviours and capabilities that inspire and support execution of a vision to deliver results. It is not used as a reference to positional authority. Furthermore, leadership should be differentiated from both governance and professionalism, although some overlap with these areas is unavoidable.

Our view of what leadership is – and what it looks like – is inevitably shaped by our expectations, exposure, education, experiences, as well as our past and current role models. Leadership is also valued differently: for some, it is a 'magic bullet' worthy of admiration and aspiration whereas others may hold a more cynical view. No matter the perception, effective leadership is as important as it has ever been.

第 1 节　为人群服务的领导力

本节将回答有关群医学领导力的六个关键问题：

- 领导力是指什么？
- 群医学中领导力的目的是什么？
- 群医学领导力有何不同？
- 群医学需要具备的关键领导力有哪些？
- 如何评价群医学领导力绩效？
- 现任领导者的角色和优先事项是什么？

■ 领导力是指什么？

> 领导力的定义不胜枚举，几乎每个尝试定义这个概念的人都会给出一个不同的定义[1]。

本书第 2 章第 3 节阐述了领导力与管理职能之间的重要区别。在此之上的进一步挑战就是如何区分领导力一词的不同用法和理解。对领导力的统一定义众说纷纭，无法达成一致。换个方式来问，就是："领导力是指什么？"

一个常见混淆点在于领导者（leader）和领导力（leadership）的使用（二者常可以互换）。在本书中，领导力一词用于描述一组基于价值观的行为和能力，可以激发并支持愿景的实施与实现。这一术语并非指职位所具有的权力。此外，领导力应与治理（governance）和职业精神（professionalism）二者区分开，尽管这些领域不可避免地有所重合。

我们对领导力的定义和看法不可避免地受到自身的期望、经历、教育、经验以及我们既往和当前榜样的影响。不同的人赋予了领导力不同的价值：对某些人来说，这是值得赞美和向往的"妙法"，而有的人觉得领导力是一个官僚主义概念，对其深感厌恶。不论人们看法如何，有效的领导力一直都非常重要。

When considering what we mean by leadership, we must also consider leadership models. A leadership model is a simplified description of a leadership system or process used to assist predictions, decisions and actions.

A common myth about leadership frequently perpetuated by medical training and practice is that leadership is by and about the individual. This myth is a consequence of narrow views on leadership that no longer apply, and it is incompatible with the new model of population medicine. An individualised view of leadership sets people apart, in a seemingly elevated and unreachable position. Adherence to this myth allows others not in a leadership position to relieve themselves of responsibility and accountability in a given situation or role, because by its very nature individualised responsibility is not shared.

This individualistic approach is compatible with a 'command and control' leadership model. The possible adverse consequences of this model include but are not limited to:

- *lack of diverse input, including the opposite view*
- *rigidity of thought*
- *disempowerment, and subsequent disengagement, of the health workforce and healthcare consumers*
- *failure to promote a positive organisational culture*

These adverse consequences and the emergence of other leadership models mean that 'command and control' is met with increasing resistance, even rejection, in the health sector and beyond. Despite this, the underlying culture of many healthcare organisations regularly reflects 'command and control' norms.

An important alternative to 'command and control' leadership is collective leadership. The King's Fund describes collective leadership as:

> *... leadership that prioritises leadership of all, by all and together with all. ... Collective leadership means leaders and teams working together across boundaries within and across organisations in the interests of patient care and community health. (2)*

Leadership and population medicine are complex; they both encompass multiple ideas, dimensions, and capabilities. To be effective and relevant to population medicine, and to attain the 'reach' required by this more integrated approach, leadership must be delivered through everyone, not merely by certain individuals with positional power. Population medicine demands collective leadership.

A possible challenge to collective leadership, as well as to similar models such as participative leadership and collaborative leadership, is the argument that

在考虑领导力的内涵时，我们还必须考虑领导模式。领导模式是对辅助预测、决策和行动的领导力体系或过程的简化描述。

关于领导力的一个常见误区是，领导力取决于个人也仅与个人有关，这一观点在医学培训和实践司空见惯并一直延续。这种观点是因过时的狭隘的领导观所致，并不能被新的群医学模式所接受。个人主义的领导观会让人脱离群众，置个人于一个看似高不可攀的位置。坚持这一错误观念就会让其他不处于领导地位的人推脱自己在特定情况或角色中的责任和义务，因为就个人主义本质而言，责任是不可分担的。

这种个人主义的方法与命令与控制领导模式相兼容。此模式可能产生的不利后果包括但不限于：

- 依靠领导个人意见行事，不去听取不同意见；
- 思想僵化；
- 医疗卫生从业人员和消费者权力的丧失及随之而来的漠不关心；
- 无法培育积极的组织文化。

这些不良后果以及其他领导模式的出现，意味着"命令与控制"模式在医疗卫生及其他部门面临越来越大的阻力，甚至遭到抗拒。尽管如此，许多医疗卫生机构的基本文化依旧以"命令与控制"模式确保日常运转。

"命令与控制"领导模式的重要替代方案是集体领导模式。国王基金会将集体领导描述为：

> ……要分清领导力是所有人共同领导还是被所有人赋予领导权或是集体领导……集体领导意味着领导者和团队为了患者照护和社区健康在机构内和机构间跨越边界进行合作[2]。

领导力和群医学都很复杂；它们都包含着多种理念、维度和功能。为了有效、有关并达到这种整合型所要求的"覆盖范围"，必须通过所有人而不仅是某些具有职位权力的人来发挥领导力作用。群医学需要集体领导模式。

集体领导模式以及类似模式——例如参与式领导和协作式领导——风险在于最终无人承担责任或义务。集体领导模式不会削弱义务感和责任感，但

no-one is ultimately responsible or accountable. Collective leadership does not diminish accountability and/or responsibility but empowers all involved to be accountable/responsible. In doing so, collective leadership places greater onus on those with positional power to be accountable to other members of the organisation and to patients.

It is also important to be explicit in stating whom leadership is for. We should be clear that our primary audience is – and must be – the population served by the health sector. With this in mind, leadership should be patient-, rather than profession-, focused, although this is not to suggest that the two are mutually exclusive.

■ What is the purpose of leadership in population medicine?

Leadership receives much attention because of the widely held view that a strong positive correlation exists between effective leadership and overall organisational performance. (3, 4) There is no better argument of the value of effective leadership than witnessing or experiencing the consequences of its absence. Signs of effective leadership, however, can remain unnoticed as an organisation ticks along partly because a key skill of those demonstrating effective leadership is to predict and address possible issues before they cause substantial problems.

In contrast, as the consequences of ineffective or poor leadership tend to penetrate multiple aspects of organisational performance, deficits in this area are difficult to hide. These consequences can range from the degree of innovation evident in organisational practices to patient satisfaction, and from staff turnover rates to the financial health and sustainability of an organisation. No matter which measure is considered, and even when only one measure is considered, it is serious.

Effective leadership is evidenced by a value-driven, safe and sustainable health system that serves the population for which it is responsible. The purpose and contribution of leadership to population medicine is inextricably linked to the purpose of population medicine itself. Owing to the absence of that message, we get caught in a fear-driven narrative that suggests leadership behaviours and actions remove us from participating in delivering care to our population, rather than promoting population care. In other words, leadership risks a reputation as a distraction rather than being perceived as critical to our central task.

The unhelpful problem of 'us and them', or worse 'us versus them', persists in the health sector. This problem directly links to and impacts on organisational and often professional culture. As leadership sets culture, the problem of 'us and them' is one of leadership.

Anecdotal evidence suggests that the 'us and them' problem is improving when it comes to the clinician–manager relationship. Despite this, divides are created and maintained in many other ways, even within relatively compact professional networks. The ethos that underpins population medicine speaks to a

能赋予所有相关人员以义务和责任心。这样做时，集体领导将更多责任下放了，由在其位者谋其政，来对机构其他成员和患者负责。

明确指出领导力的目标人群也很重要的。我们应当清楚，我们的主要受众是——而且必须是——医疗卫生保健部门所关注的人群。考虑到这一点，领导力应该以患者为中心，而非以职业为中心，但这并不意味着两者互斥。

■ 群医学中领导力的目的是什么？

领导力受到了广泛关注是因为人们普遍认为有效领导力与组织总体绩效之间存在很强的正相关[3, 4]。证明有效领导力价值的最好方式就是目睹或经历领导力缺乏导致的后果。然而，机构发展顺利时，有效领导力的作用可能会被忽视，部分原因在于有此才能的人的关键本领就是预见尚未出现的实际问题并在其导致不良后果出现前解决它。

相反，无效或不良领导力的后果往往会通过机构绩效的多个方面表现出来，因此很难掩盖。后果可能表现在从医疗卫生机构工作实践的创新程度到患者满意度，也可能表现在员工流动率、财务状况的健康性和可持续性等多个方面。无论出现哪个方面问题，其后果都很严重，即使仅出现其中一种后果。

有效领导力体现在以价值为导向、安全和可持续的医疗卫生保健体系中，该系统对接受其医疗的人群负责。领导力在群医学中应用的目的和对其的贡献与群医学本身目的密不可分。由于缺少以上信息，我们陷入了恐惧驱动的叙事中，该叙事形式认为领导力行为和行动会使我们脱离而不是促进人群的医疗照护。换句话说，这种领导行为要冒被误解的风险，大家会认为这对于实现核心任务是干扰而非关键之举。

"我们与他们"或更糟糕的"我们与他们相比"等无益问题仍然持续存在于医疗卫生部门。这个问题与机构文化（通常还有职业文化）直接挂钩并产生影响。当领导力在设置文化时，"我们与他们"的问题便是领导力内容之一。

坊间证据表明，临床医生与管理者之间，"我们与他们"的问题正在改善。尽管如此，就算专业工作网络联系相对紧密，依然有许多其他方式产生分歧并长期存在。群医学的基本理念代表一种承诺，即找出并解决那些产生

commitment to identify and address factors that build and/or preserve unnecessary and artificial divisions. A continued focus on the purpose of leadership in population medicine brings us back to common ground, which is the platform for progress.

■ What is different about leadership in population medicine?

The temptation is to consider that we need a different niche approach to leadership for different sectors, or even different areas within sectors.

Population medicine, and indeed health, is not special but it is different. Although specific details will differ and appropriate tailoring will always be required, the fundamental principles and challenges of leadership remain consistent and largely transferable across multiple sectors, such as education and the military. (5, 6) There is greater risk in narrowing our thinking and skill set, under the pretence of enhanced specialisation, to a level that limits our ability to adapt and appropriately respond to new, unpredictable challenges.

Nonetheless, we must be explicit in stating that strong clinician involvement is a requirement for effective leadership in population medicine. This is no different from leadership requirements elsewhere in the health domain.

Although clinicians are not the sole stewards of population medicine, the value and unique contribution of clinical leaders and clinical leadership are well recognised.

Another important qualification is that we have to be clear and careful about how we think about and deploy leadership in the context of population medicine. Continuing to support or demonstrate outdated and ineffective leadership serves no-one. Therefore, we move from the original question of how leadership in population medicine might differ from leadership deployed elsewhere to ask instead 'What needs to be different about our existing leadership practices and behaviours to move toward a population medicine approach successfully?'

We must turn to best thinking and practice and, in doing so, refer back to the collective leadership model outlined above. Just as population medicine shifts attention from one patient to the population with a given condition, leadership in population medicine requires that we shift our view from that of the stand- alone leader to consider leadership behaviours and capabilities that are collectively displayed by a team working together and sharing responsibility and accountability for the delivery of common goals.

■ What are the leadership requirements in population medicine?

Effective leadership in population medicine will occur only if there is sustained, deliberate investment in leadership development. We outline eight high-level principles to guide leadership development for those engaged in population medicine.

- *First, leadership development should employ a values-based approach. (7) A key challenge in medicine has always been the inherent uncertainty associated with healthcare journeys, both at the individual and population levels.*

和 / 或留存的不必要人为分歧的因素。继续关注群医学领导力的目的可以把我们带回共同点，这是取得进步的平台。

■ 群医学所需的领导力有何不同？

我们常常觉得需要针对不同行业甚至行业内不同领域来采用不同方法实现领导力。

群医学（实际上是整个医疗卫生保健行业）与其他行业相比，并非特别但也有所差异。尽管具体细节不同且始终需要适当调整，但是不同行业（如教育和军事）的领导力的基本原则和挑战仍然是一致的，并且可以互相借鉴[5, 6]。然而，在加强专业化的借口下，我们的思维和技能变得狭隘的风险更大。这限制了我们适应和应对新的、不可预测的挑战的能力。

但是，我们必须明确指出，临床医生的大力参与是实现群医学所需有效领导力的必要条件。这与医疗卫生保健行业其他领域的领导力要求并无二致。尽管临床医生不是群医学的唯一管理者，但临床领导者和临床领导力的价值和独特贡献已得到公认。

在群医学的背景下，我们如何看待和调配领导力？保持明智谨慎是另一个重要的限定条件。继续支持或证实领导力过时无效对任何人都没有好处。因此，我们将最初的问题"群医学与其他领域中调动的领导力有何不同"替换为"要成功地迈向群医学模式，我们现有领导力的实践和行为应做何转变？"

我们必须向最佳思维和实践转变，并在行动时参考上面提及的集体领导模式。正如群医学将注意力从个体患者转向某些特定患病人群一样，群医学要求我们转变观念，从独立领导者转变为由团队集体领导，以及为实现共同目标分担责任义务的领导行为和能力。

■ 群医学需要具备的领导力有哪些？

只有持续主动地投入，才能在群医学领域发挥有效领导力。我们列出了八项高级指导原则，让从事群医学工作的人们发展领导力。

• 第一，发展领导力应采用基于价值观的方法[7]。医学上的一个主要挑战一直是个人和人群医疗。

Leadership needs to be guided by values to navigate this uncertainty, and to be seen as authentic. Leadership values should be defined locally to align with organisational values, some of which are provided below.

Integrity	Service	Respect
Courage	Compassion	Curiosity
Resilience	Self-awareness	Excellence

- *Second, leadership development initiatives require visible, high-level sponsorship at both local and national levels. This support asserts the role and importance of leadership in population medicine.*
- *Third, leadership capability should be developed across the workforce engaged in designing and delivering population medicine.*
- *The fourth principle is that leadership development is a long-term process. A long-term approach requires the vision to invest in those at relatively early career stages. This means that the identification, recruitment and development of future leaders are issues that demand attention and action now. Importantly, this investment must accompany and not replace development opportunities for those with current positional authority.*
- *Fifth, opportunities for leadership development should reflect what is known about how leadership development occurs. Models such as the 70/20/10 model (see Figure 3.1) for learning and development are helpful references. A cursory examination of this pyramid reminds us that experiential learning opportunities should form the basis of leadership development journeys. Furthermore, these experiences should occur in real work settings. (8)*
- *Sixth, technical expertise must be distinguished from leadership ability. A common scenario in healthcare organisations is that people are offered positions with considerable leadership responsibility based on their proven technical expertise in a certain area. This technical expertise is assumed to translate into effective performance in a very different role. Leadership ability and technical prowess, however, are not necessarily correlated; dedicated leadership development is relevant to everyone irrespective of role or positioning in the sector.*
- *Seventh, inter-disciplinary approaches to leadership development are to be encouraged. Among other benefits, inter-disciplinary learning promotes a 'collective team identity' (9), which aligns with a collective leadership model.*
- *Last but not least, evaluation is integral to good practice and should be incorporated into all leadership development activity.*

卫生保健过程中的内在不确定性。领导力需要以价值观为指导以消除这种不确定性，并被视为真实存在的。领导力相关价值观应根据当地情况确定并与机构的价值观保持一致，其中一些常见价值观如下：

诚信	服务	尊重
勇气	慈悲	求知
韧性	自省	卓越

- 第二，领导力发展计划需要得到地方和国家两个层面的明确高度支持。这种支持肯定了群医学中领导力的作用和重要性。
- 第三，应该培养所有参与构建和实施群医学工作人员的领导能力。
- 第四，领导力发展是一个长期过程。长期发展模式需要远见，投资于职场新人而非老手。这意味着甄选、招募和培养未来领导者需要马上关注并采取行动。重要的是，这项投入必须伴随而非取代当前管理人员的发展机会。
- 第五，领导力发展机会应该反映出人们对领导力培养过程的理解。用于学习和发展的模型便是有用的参考，例如 70/20/10 模型（图 3.1）。对这个金字塔的初步分析提醒我们，积累经验的学习机会应构成领导力发展过程的基础。此外，这些经验应该在实际的工作环境中积累[8]。
- 第六，必须将技术专长与领导能力相区分。在医疗卫生机构中，常见的情况是，根据职员在某个领域展示出的技术专长为其提供重要责任的职位。这种技术专长被假定可以转变去有效履行另一个不同角色的职能。但是，领导能力和技术能力并不一定相关。致力于领导力发展与每个人都息息相关，无论其在行业中的角色或定位如何。
- 第七，鼓励采用跨学科方法发展领导力。除其他好处外，跨学科学习还促进了"集体团队身份"的形成[9]，并与集体领导模式保持一致。
- 最后但也是同样重要的一项是，评估为良好实践的组成部分，应将其纳入所有领导力发展活动中。

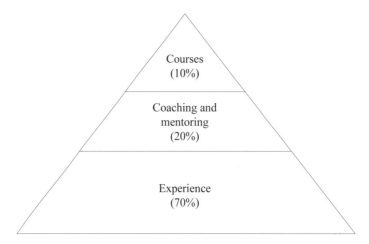

Figure 3.1   Learning and Development Model (adapted from reference 10)

These high-level principles speak to how leadership development should be approached. The next step is to determine what should actually be developed. There is no definitive checklist for leadership development and a discussion of the relative merits of various leadership capabilities lies beyond the scope of this book but four requirements for leadership in population medicine warrant special mention:

- *adaptability*
- *resilience*
- *courage*
- *diversity*

These capabilities are not typically taught in a classroom situation.

In considering the requirements for leadership in population medicine, we also reflect on the role and importance of time. A common mistake is to assume that leadership is reserved for those at later career stages. We know, however, that leadership is not defined by role. We have also established that collective leadership necessitates an inclusive approach. Furthermore, time offers no guarantees. Time is often a valuable asset in leadership development, but the process still requires deliberate attention and action. A lack of time, which may or may not translate into a lack of experience, does not necessarily preclude the presence of leadership behaviours and capabilities. Certain leadership capabilities, such as building teams and thinking and acting strategically, are more likely to be present in those with considerable experience in a certain role or area. Other leadership capabilities, however, can be, and often are, demonstrated by those at relatively early career stages. Finally, more time is not always better: the youth are on the battlefield first because they can run the fastest. We must move toward a situation where the particular capabilities and strengths of the range of individuals are recognised and used appropriately.

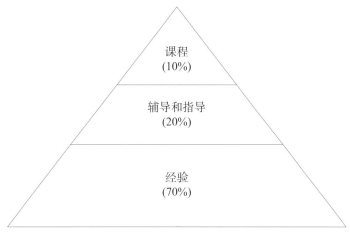

图 3.1　学习与发展模型（改编自参考文献 10）

这些高级别原则说明了如何实现领导力。下一步是明确应该培养哪些领导力。领导力发展没有明确清单，各种领导能力优缺点的讨论也不在本书的范围之内，但需要特别提及群医学领域的四个领导力要求：

- 适应性；
- 韧性；
- 勇气；
- 多元化。

这些能力通常不会在课堂上传授。

在考虑群医学的领导力要求时，我们还反思了时间的作用和重要性。一个常见的错误认知是领导力专指职场高层人员。然而，我们知道领导力不是由职业角色定义的。还可以肯定的是，集体领导必须采取包容性方法。此外，时间不是获得领导力的保证。时间通常是领导力发展中的宝贵资产，但是能力的发展过程仍然需要主动关注和行动。缺乏时间投入（可能会或不会导致经验缺乏）并不一定会妨碍领导行为和能力的存在。在某些职位或领域具有丰富经验的人员更有可能具有特定领导能力，例如建设团队和策划采取战略行动。然而，职场菜鸟也可能且经常展示出其他领导能力。最后，时间更多并非总是更好：年轻人打头阵是因为他们跑得快。我们必须营造这么一种环境——每个个体的特定能力和优势可以在其中得到认可和适当发挥。

■ How do we measure leadership performance in population medicine?

Measuring leadership performance in population medicine is a complex process. Before considering how leadership should be assessed, it is worth examining the current processes and associated issues.

There is no shortage of frameworks for leadership and leadership development. Leadership attributes and/or capabilities are now commonly defined; many are even tailored to organisational priorities and different roles and/or career levels, however, gaps in knowledge remain. For example, how do we measure against these frameworks in a valid and reliable fashion? In the context of ever-changing broader environments and rapid, cross-sectional review cycles, we are limited because it is not possible to link isolated inputs to observed long-term outcomes.

Also, in many instances, leadership frameworks themselves are unproven. The frameworks may well be grounded in established theory and evidence, but the outcomes of applying a framework to leadership are not always clear. This could be because the outcomes are not formally considered or articulated, or because outcomes are of uncertain relevance.

There are at least three further issues associated with current processes for measuring leadership performance that merit attention. First, leadership is generally assessed against a pre-defined, inflexible cluster of behaviours or skills that have little relevance to a person's role or to organisational requirements. Worse still, the behaviours or skills may have little or no relevance to health outcomes, let alone to the broader system. Assessments of leadership performance conducted using inappropriate measures are unlikely to guide and support future improvements. Instead, they may simply fuel frustration in those tasked with delivering care to populations who seek to assess and improve their effectiveness.

Second, under the old paradigm in healthcare, the default has been to assess performance at an individual level based on specific, isolated measures that link to a single medical specialty or condition. This approach may be helpful, but it is not sufficient; it takes little account of the overall environment in which the measures are produced. Typically, this approach also neglects to identify trade-offs involved in generating particular measures.

Third, the current system risks a situation whereby certain individual-level leadership attributes, such as general likeability or confidence, are confused with leadership potential and/or performance. Indeed, there is an inverse relationship between overconfidence and leadership potential and/or performance. Indeed, there is an inverse relationship between overconfidence and leadership performance. (11) Progress toward a common understanding of what is meant by leadership in population medicine can help to minimise such confusion but will not disguise the need for a more comprehensive, systematic approach to measurement of leadership performance. Such an approach, grounded in the principles of collective leadership, requires trust.

■ 如何评价群医学领导力的绩效？

评估群医学领导力的绩效是一个复杂的过程。在考虑如何评估领导力之前，有必要检查当前的工作流程和相关问题。

当前不缺领导力和领导力发展的框架。现在领导力的属性和 / 或能力已被广泛定义；许多甚至是根据组织的优先事项和不同岗位角色和 / 或职业水平量身定制；但是，认识方面的差距仍然存在。例如，我们如何以有效可靠的方式评估这些框架？环境越变越广泛，评审周期时间短跨度大，在此种背景下，我们不可能将单独的投入与观察到的长期结果联系起来，因此备受局限。

同样，在许多情况下，领导力框架本身未经证实。框架很可能建立在既定的理论和证据上，但是将框架应用于领导力的结果并不总是明确的。这可能是由于未对结果进行正式审议或明确表达，或者是由于结果的相关性不确定。

当前评估领导力绩效的过程还有至少三个问题值得关注。首先，领导力通常根据预先定义的、很少变化的行为或技能来评估，而这些与个人的岗位角色或组织要求无关。更糟糕的是，这些行为或技能可能与健康结果几乎无关，遑论更广泛的医疗卫生保健体系。使用不当指标评估领导力绩效评估难以指导并支持未来的改进。相反，它们可能只增强了那些希望通过评估提高效率的医护人员的挫败感。

其次，在旧有医疗卫生保健范式下，通常根据特定的、与单个专科或疾病相关的独立指标来评估个人绩效。这种方法可能是适宜的，但还有缺陷：它很少考虑设计这些评估措施的总体环境。通常，此方法也忽略了对生成特定评价指标的权衡取舍。

第三，当前的评价体系面临着这样一种风险，即某些个体的领导力属性（例如亲和力或自信心）会与领导力潜能和 / 或绩效相混淆。确实，过度自信与领导力绩效之间呈反比关系[11]。对群医学领导力的涵义达成共识可以帮助最大程度地减少这种混淆，但不会掩盖对领导力绩效的更全面、系统化评估方法的需求。这种基于集体领导原则的评估方法需要信任。

Ultimately leadership performance will be measured and defined by the performance of the system. In the context of population medicine, this means outcomes that display value and sustainability at the population level, together with the minimisation of waste, suffering and other harm. Further principles to help guide evaluation of leadership in population medicine are listed below.

- *The principal audience for the evaluation should not differ from the principal audience for population medicine, that is, the population served by the health sector*
- *Measures must include both short- and long-term outcomes*
- *Measures must demonstrate direct alignment with organisational values and goals*
- *Evaluation findings should be placed in the context of the wider environment and include information about external influences (e.g. political priorities), possible confounders and recent trends*
- *The evaluation should incorporate evaluation of the framework/approach itself*

Finally, it is important to note that a system-level approach does not negate the need for evaluation of individuals or single areas/projects. Instead, comprehensive measurement of leadership performance should incorporate assessment conducted by self, other staff, the population served (e.g. patient satisfaction and patient-reported outcome measures), and members of the governance board.

■ What are the roles and priorities of current leaders?

Current leaders have several priority tasks as we move toward a population-medicine approach.

First, current leaders should commit to moving beyond narrow, individualistic leadership models to adopt collective leadership. This model enables an organisation to address the complex challenges of population medicine by applying diverse yet complementary knowledge, experience, skills and attributes, and by empowering staff to achieve shared goals.

Second, leaders must define and communicate their vision around the purpose and contribution of population medicine. The role of leadership in population medicine should be directly aligned with this vision and positioned as critical to the task. Current leaders must also articulate their vision of the nature of success, and the specific measures against which success will be determined.

Another priority task is for current leaders to work collectively to establish the leadership values that will guide and underpin future work in population medicine. (12) It is incumbent on all leaders to ensure that these values are demonstrated in routine decisions and actions, and to foster an organisational culture that supports their widespread application. This latter role incorporates recognising where values are demonstrated, and appropriately highlighting and responding to actions and/or behaviours that are inconsistent with agreed values.

最终，领导力绩效将由医疗卫生保健体系的绩效来衡量和定义。在群医学的背景下，这意味着在人群水平展现出有价值和可持续性的成果，同时将浪费、痛苦和其他危害降至最低。下面列出了有助于指导评估群医学领导力的进阶原则：

- 评估的主要对象不应与群医学的主要对象（即接受医疗人群）不同；
- 评估指标必须包括短期和长期结果；
- 评估指标必须直接对标组织的价值观和目标；
- 评价结果应放在更广泛的环境中进行解读，并应包括有关外部影响的信息（例如政治优先事项）、可能的混杂因素和近期趋势；
- 评估应纳入对评价框架/方法本身的评估。

最后，值得注意的是，系统层面的评估方法并非否定评估个人或单个领域/项目的需要。而是说对领导力绩效的全面评估应纳入以下人员：自身、其他员工、接受医疗的人群（例如患者满意度和患者报告结果等指标）及治理委员会成员等。

■ 现任领导者的角色和优先事项是什么？

在向群医学模式发展时，现任领导人有数项优先任务。

首先，现任领导者应致力于超越狭隘的个人主义领导模式，实行集体领导。该模式使组织能够通过应用各种互补知识、经验、技能和属性来应对群医学的复杂挑战，并赋予员工权力以实现共同的目标。

其次，领导者必须围绕群医学的目的和作用来定义和传达他们的愿景。群医学中领导力的角色应与这一愿景直接挂钩，也是实现愿景的关键。现任领导人还必须阐明对成功本质的看法以及决定成功所需采取的具体评估措施。

当前领导者的另一项优先任务是共同努力，建立领导力价值观以指导和支持未来的群医学工作[12]。所有领导者都有责任确保在日常决策和行动中体现这些价值观，并培养支持其广泛应用的组织文化。后者角色包括认识到这些价值观应在何处呈现，并适当地强调与商定价值观不一致的行动和/或行为，且做出响应。

To execute any strategy for population medicine, current leaders must be equipped with apposite knowledge of: population medicine itself; the health condition(s); the population served; available resource (including staff experience and capability); and other factors that may impact on delivery of any future strategy, such as emerging or competing priorities. Here, integrity, insight and courage are required to recognise and address any current knowledge gaps.

Lastly, current leaders in population medicine have a vested interest in supporting and encouraging others to live up to their potential. Therefore, supporting leadership development and deployment must always rank amongst the highest of organisational priorities.

■ Questions for reflection

- *What is the predominant leadership model in your organisation? What is needed to move toward collective leadership?*
- *What are the leadership values of your organisation?*
- *How does your organisation define successful leadership?*
- *How is leadership recognised and incentivised in your organisation?*
- *How is the development of future leadership being actively encouraged and supported in your organisation? How could you contribute to this process?*
- *How is diversity in leadership promoted and maintained in your organisation?*

References

(1) Stogdill RM. Handbook of leadership: A survey of theory and research. New York: The Free Press; 1974: 259.

(2) West M. Collective leadership: fundamental to creating the cultures we need in the NHS. Kings Fund Website. www.kingsfund.org.uk. Updated May 21, 2014. Accessed July 21, 2014.

(3) Hogan R, Kaiser RB. What we know about leadership. Review of General Psychology. 2005; 9(2): 169-180.

(4) Collins J. Good to great. New York: Harper Collins; 2001.

(5) Pinnington AH. Leadership development: Applying the same leadership theories and development practices to different contexts? Leadership. 2011; 7(3): 335-365.

(6) Gentry WA, Eckert RH, Stawiski SA, Zhao S. The challenges leaders face around the world: More similar than different. Center for Creative Leadership, White Paper. 2014.

(7) O'Toole J. Leading change: The argument for values-based leadership. New York:

要执行任何群医学战略，现任领导者必须具备以下恰当知识：群医学；健康状况；接受医疗的人群；可用资源（包括员工经验和能力）以及可能影响实施任何未来战略的其他因素，例如新出现的或彼此冲突的优先事项。因此，需要有正直、洞察力和勇气来正视和解决当前的任何知识不足。

最后，当前的群医学领导者也会受益了支持和鼓励他人发挥自己的潜力。因此，支持领导力的发展和部署必须始终处于组织工作的重中之重。

■ 思考题

- 机构或组织中主要的领导模式是什么？要实现集体领导需要什么？

- 机构的领导力价值观是什么？

- 机构如何定义成功的领导力？

- 如何在机构中认可和激励领导力？

- 如何在机构中积极鼓励和支持未来领导力的发展？您如何为这一过程做出贡献？

- 如何在机构中促进和维持领导力的多样性？

参考文献

Ballantine Books; 1996.

(8) Gurdjian P, Halbeisen T, Lane K. Why leadership-development programs fail. McKinsey Quarterly Website www.mckinsey.com/insights/leading_in_the_21st_century. Updated January 2014. Accessed July 21, 2014.

(9) Willis D. Emerging leaders: learning together to deliver future health care. The Kings Fund Website www.kingsfund.org.uk/blog/2014/03/emerging-leaders-learning- together-deliver-future-health-care. Accessed April 2014. Updated July 21, 2014.

(10) Lombardo MM, Eichinger RW. The Career Architect Development Planner. 1st Edition. Minneapolis: Lominger; 2000.

(11) Shipman AS, Mumford MD. When confidence is detrimental: Influence of overconfidence on leadership effectiveness. The Leadership Quarterly. 2011; 22(4): 649-665.

(12) Bennis W. The challenges of leadership in the modern world. American Psychologist. 2007; 62(1): 1-5.

3.2 Quality improvement that serves populations

In this section, we explore:

- *'quality' and 'quality improvement'*
- *actions that can be taken to protect and improve quality*
- *where to start in relation to 'System and resources'*
- *where to start in relation to 'Performance monitoring and re-adjustment'*
- *how to engage the system in Continuous Quality Improvement*
- *healthcare quality*
- *how healthcare improvement can contribute to the practice of population medicine*

■ How do we accelerate and expand quality improvement?

Quality and quality improvement seem to have been constantly in the healthcare news. A simple Google search of 'quality healthcare' brings up 141 million hits. On the international stage, there has been the high-profile 'Mid Staffs' enquiry, followed by numerous other investigations into 'poor quality care' at institutions around the world. Don Berwick chaired The National Advisory Group for the Safety of Patients in England (A Promise to Learn – A Commitment to Act) and the executive summary on the website begins:

> *Place the quality of patient care, especially patient safety, above all other aims. (1)*

At the same time, healthcare services the world over face multiple challenges, not least fiscal issues, coupled with corridor conversations that indicate many senior executives still see quality as something of a luxury.

So how do we accelerate important quality improvement work? How do we extend the learning and the vision from a hospital focus to a whole-of-system and whole-of-population one?

A key component of positive change will be to develop a common understanding and a common language, with recognition of the common underlying philosophy and methodology.

第 2 节　为提升人群服务的质量

在本章节中，我们将探讨：

• "质量"和"质量改善"；

• 保护和改善质量可采取的行动；

• 如何从"系统与资源"的角度入手；

• 从何处开始"绩效监测和重新调整"；

• 如何在系统中引入"持续性质量改善"；

• 医疗卫生保健的质量；

• 医疗卫生保健的改善如何促进群医学实践。

■ 我们如何加快并扩展质量改善？

质量和质量改善似乎频频出现在医疗卫生保健相关新闻中。如果我们在谷歌上搜索关键词"优质医疗卫生保健"，会得到 1.41 亿条结果。国际上曾经有过备受关注的"医疗人员"调查，随之又有大量在世界各地医疗机构中对"劣质医疗卫生保健"的调查。

唐·贝里克是英格兰国家患者安全咨询小组的主席，他的报告《言必行，行必果》在网站上摘要的开头这样写道：

将患者照护质量——尤其是患者安全——作为医疗卫生服务的首要目的[1]。

与此同时，全球医疗卫生保健在实现此目标时面临着诸多挑战，不仅是财政问题，许多高层管理人员在访谈时也曾表示医疗的高质量千金难求。

那么，我们如何加快如此重要的质量改善工作呢？又如何将关注点和视野从医院扩展到聚焦整个卫生体系和整个人群呢？

积极改变的一个关键组成部分是发展共识和共同语言，以及对共同哲学思想和方法论的认知。

Therefore, in this section, we review some of the core elements of quality improvement, and the assurance of quality, with a population view.

The challenge and some ground rules

The care we would be happy for our families and our communities to experience is dependent on Continuous Quality Improvement, as well as the important assurance functions that hold and demonstrate the gains.

The challenge for those interested in population medicine, as for colleagues leading individual patient care, is 'establishing, protecting, promoting and improving' quality. Donabedian gives three important pieces of advice as we face this challenge. (2)

1.Understand, maintain, and improve quality: As healthcare professionals, we must understand the quality of the care we provide and strive to maintain and to improve that quality.

2.Do not be seduced by 'new methods' or fads: 'the new is, many times,

… mostly a continuation of the old … what seems shiningly new is no more than a reinvention of the formerly known, perhaps with an added emphasis or twist, or possibly under a new, more alluring, name.' (3) This is important for us to hold onto when we struggle with the multiplicity of 'methodologies'

3.Expand your view to all levels of the system: The advent of Total Quality Management has helped to expand the scope of quality improvement work from individual care provided by practitioners to every activity within a healthcare organisation, and now such continual improvement work needs to take a whole-of-population view

Defining and designing Continuous Quality Improvement (CQI)

Donabedian defines quality improvement in a way that both describes a whole-of-population view and embraces the elements of quality assurance, quality improvement and quality control found in many other definitions or schools of quality.

All actions taken to establish, protect, promote and improve the quality of healthcare. (4)

Very appropriately for a population, Continuous Quality Improvement (CQI) as envisaged by Donabedian, can be divided into two parts. (2)

1.System and resources: recognises that the 'design' must promote, not obstruct, good care, and that resources must be sufficient. Design includes elements of professional recruitment, education, training and certification of staff

因此，在本节中，我们将从人群角度审视质量改善和质量保障的一些核心要素。

挑战和基本原则

我们乐意让家人和社区享受的医疗照护依赖于持续性质量改善（CQI）以及重要保障功能，以保持和证明质量改进所取得的成果。

一些对群医学感兴趣的医疗从业人员（如引领个体患者照护的同行）所面临的挑战便是"建立、保护、促进并改善"医疗卫生质量。唐·贝里克针对挑战给出了三条重要建议[2]。

1. 理解、维护并改善医疗质量：作为医疗卫生专业人员，我们必须了解我们提供照护的质量，并努力维护和改善质量。

2. 不要痴迷"新方法""新潮流"："所谓的'新'，很多时候……主要是'旧'的延续……那些看起来光彩夺目的新事物，不过是对旧事物的改造——或强化或转化某些已有功能，或仅是披上一个新的、更诱人的名字[3]。"认识到这点有助于我们在面对琳琅满目的"方法论"时坚持正确的选择。

3. 将视野拓展到系统的各个层面：全面质量管理的出现有助于将质量改善工作的范围从由个体医疗照护扩展到医疗卫生保健机构中的各项活动中。现在，我们需要从全人群角度持续开展医疗质量的改善工作。

持续性质量改善（CQI）的定义和设计

多纳贝迪安既从全人群的角度定义了医疗卫生质量的改善，也包含了其他定义和学派中关于质量保障、质量改善和质量控制的元素。

> 为建立、保护、促进和改善医疗卫生保健质量而采取的所有措施[4]。

多纳贝迪安所设想的 CQI 非常适用于人群，它可以分为两部分[2]：

1. 系统和资源：认识到"设计"目的必须是促进而不是阻碍优质医疗照护，且相应资源也必须充足。设计应涵盖招聘专业人才、教育、培训和员工认证等要素。

2.Performance monitoring and re-adjustment: relates to obtaining information about the level of quality produced by the health system, based on interpretation of that information, and taking action to protect and improve quality

Many descriptions of quality improvement gloss over system design and system resources. In these situations, there is a singular focus on the second part of Donabedian's equation, because monitoring and re-adjustment are perceived as more amenable to action. Sadly, we can see internationally the consequences of reduced training and quality improvement budgets.

Investment in education and quality improvement is crucial in the achievement of a high-performing organisation, and it becomes even more important when organisations face challenges that must be overcome by finding better, more efficient ways of providing care.

What sort of actions can one take to protect and improve quality?

Continuous Quality Improvement is the basis of many quality improvement methodologies, such as Plan Do Study Act (PDSA), the Model for Improvement, Plan Do Check Act (PDCA) and Six Sigma. Observation, interpretation, action and assessment are key principles applied in the CQI process.

Where to start? System and resources

In considering 'system and resources', there is an opportunity to educate and motivate people within your organisation, and partner organisations. Train together, build networks, build collaborative projects. Bring leadership from partner organisations together to review progress. Working with system resources in this way is difficult, but it was a key driver for the establishment of the Centre for Improvement, Ko Awatea, in Counties Manukau District Health Board, New Zealand. Our belief was that by building a career pipeline that engaged talent in our local community, by ensuring our workforce reflected our local community, by making our health system engaging to learn within, and by surrounding all undergraduate and postgraduate education with improvement and innovation activity, we would build the motivated, educated workforce needed to deliver the highest quality services.

Working at a population level to improve the design of training and to resource the system that produces our staff, we believe will improve the performance of healthcare workers and reduce the potential for unwarranted variation.

Where to start? Performance monitoring and re-adjustment

There are two types of monitoring: informal and formal. Informal monitoring can take many forms, but quality tends to increase as practitioners work together through collaborative work, multidisciplinary meetings, clinical rounds, and so on. In contrast, when individual practitioners work in isolation, it is difficult to identify

2. 绩效监测和重新调整：此内容涉及获取医疗系统质量水平的相关信息，基于信息解读并采取措施保护和改善医疗质量。

质量改善的描述鲜有提及系统设计和系统资源。在这些情况下，人们把焦点仅放在多纳贝迪安等式的第二部分，因为监测和重新调整比行动更容易感知。遗憾的是，我们可以从国际上看到减少培训和质量改善预算带来的后果。

一个组织或机构要想实现高效运作，投资教育和质量改善至关重要；当组织必须通过寻找更好更有效的医疗卫生照护提供方式来克服这些挑战时，这一点就变得更加重要。

我们可以采取什么行动来保护和改善质量？

CQI 是许多质量改善方法论的基础，例如计划 – 执行 – 学习 – 处理法（PDSA）、质量改善模型、计划 – 行动检查 – 改善法（PDCA）和六西格玛法[①] 等。观察、解释、行动和评估是应用 CQI 流程中的关键原则。

从何处入手？系统及资源

考虑到"系统和资源"，组织内部及合作组织中有机会教育和激励人们，让他们一起参与培训，建立工作网络，开展协作项目。同时也可以召集各组织领导一起审核进展情况。以这种方式利用系统资源固然存在困难，但也不乏先例，例如新西兰马考努卫生局便是借鉴此方法建立了寇·阿瓦提创新与改进研究所。这背后传达的理念是，我们通过建立"定向医疗卫生保健人员培养项目"吸引本地人才并确保人才尽用，将改进和创新的概念引入所有本科和研究生教育，从而建立一支积极进取且受过良好教育的、能够提供高质量医疗的员工队伍。

在群体层面改善培训设计并丰富人力建设资源，有助于提高医疗卫生人员的绩效并保持稳定。

从何处入手？绩效监测和重新调整

绩效监测可分两种类型：非正式和正式。非正式监测可采用多种形式，但是随着医生通过协作、多学科会议、临床查房等合作加强，质量会趋于提

---

① 六西格码（Six Sigma）：一种改善企业质量流程管理的技术。

optimal practice.

It is also important to establish formal monitoring processes that are uniformly implemented, predictable and acceptable.

Engaging the system in CQI

It is not possible to undertake quality improvement, or any of its component parts, including quality monitoring, without a willingness to engage. Most important of all is a team commitment to quality.

Both the commitment to quality and the development of a mechanism to monitor quality relies on an agreed definition of quality. Once quality has been defined, there is an opportunity to engage staff and patients in the pursuit of safety, or other domains of quality. Standards, once developed, lend themselves to audit cycles, which can be used to engage junior and senior healthcare staff and teams.

1: Define healthcare quality

There are many definitions of healthcare quality. The Institute of Medicine (IOM) has proposed one that captures the features of many other definitions and which has received wide acceptance.

> *The degree to which health services for individuals and populations increase the likelihood of desired health outcomes and are consistent with current professional knowledge. (5)*

As encompassing as that definition is, it does not provide much guidance to a researcher interested in developing a measure or set of measures. A subsequent IOM report specified six aims for a high-quality medical care system that are more specific (6):

- *Safe – avoiding injuries to patients from the care that is supposed to help them*
- *Effective – providing services based on scientific knowledge to all who could benefit and refraining from providing services to those not likely to benefit (avoiding under-use and over-use)*
- *Patient-centred – providing care that is respectful of and responsive to individual patient preferences, needs, and values, and ensuring that patient values guide all clinical decisions*
- *Timely – reducing waits and sometimes harmful delays for both those who receive and those who give care*
- *Efficient – avoiding waste, in particular waste of equipment, supplies, ideas, and energy*

高。相反，当医生以孤立方式工作时，我们将很难确定最佳实践①。

当然，建立统一实施、可预测且可接受的正式监测流程也很重要。

将系统引入 CQI

如果团队没有参与意愿，就不可能开展包括质量监测在内的质量改善或其子项目。团队对质量的承诺重于一切。

对质量的承诺和质量监测机制的发展都需要先对医疗质量形成一个统一定义。一旦有了明确的医疗质量定义，我们在追求安全性或其他质量领域目标时，便可让员工和患者参与其中。相关标准一旦制定，就可以纳入评审过程，让初级和资深医疗卫生人员与团队参与进来。

1. 定义医疗服务质量

医疗服务质量存在诸多定义。美国医学研究所（IOM）提出了一种囊括多种定义特征的版本并已得到广泛认可。

> 为个体和群体提供医疗照护的程度可以提升预期健康结果并与现有专业知识相一致[5]。

尽管这个定义包罗万象，它对于想要制定一项或多项评估措施的研究人员而言并无太多指导意义。由此，IOM 提出了更为明确的高质量医疗卫生照护体系的六个目标[6]：

- 安全——医疗服务旨在帮助患者，因此在服务过程中应避免患者受到伤害；
- 有效——向所有受益者提供基于科学知识的医疗，并避免向不大可能受益的人提供医疗（以避免资源使用不足和过度使用）；
- 以患者为中心——在提供医疗卫生保健时尊重患者的个人偏好、需求和价值观，并考虑患者价值观以指导所有临床决策；
- 及时——减少医疗提供方和接受方的等待时间和延误；
- 高效——避免浪费，尤其是设备、耗材、想法和精力方面的浪费；

---

① 最佳实践（best practice）：管理学概念，认为存在某种技术、方法、过程、活动或机制可以使生产或管理实践的结果达到最优，并减少出错的可能性。

- *Equitable – providing care that does not vary in quality because of personal characteristics, such as gender, ethnicity, geographic location, and socio-economic status*

Others have also produced important definitions of quality. (7)

We propose defining it as the combined and unceasing efforts of everyone—healthcare professionals, patients and their families, researchers, payers, planners and educators—to make the changes that will lead to better patient outcomes (health), better system performance (care) and better professional development.

Donabedian, in many ways the founder of the healthcare quality movement, said in a lecture that:

... the quality of a health service is the degree to which it conforms to pre-set standards of goodness. (8)

2: Set three levels of standard

When setting standards, it is important to be aware that standards are subjective, and different perspectives exist. A manager may think a service is of good quality, but patients and carers may regard its quality as poor, or vice versa. Many people rate their experience with alternative or complementary medicine as high in quality, whereas many clinicians would regard such services as low in value.

It is often useful to set more than one level of standard. In a book popular in the 1990s entitled In Search of Excellence (9), people were exhorted to be excellent. Unfortunately, exhortations to excellence can be de-motivating for people working in difficult circumstances aware that excellence is the result not only of hard work, but often of the chance coalition of skilful individuals working in a propitious environment. For this reason, it is advisable to set three levels of standard:

- *a minimal acceptable standard, below which no programme of care should fall*
- *an excellent standard, which is attained by the best services*
- *an achievable standard, for example, the cut-off point between the top quartile of service performance and the remainder of services*

3: Engage through monitoring clinical performance

Most monitoring is either externally required or internally motivated. Externally required monitoring is a fact of life: it is necessary to provide assurance to the prevailing bureaucracy. Internally motivated monitoring has considerable

- 公平——提供的医疗质量不因人而异（例如性别、种族、地理位置和社会经济地位）。

其他学者也提出了医疗质量的重要定义[7]。

　　我们建议对医疗卫生服务质量做出如下定义：所有参与者（医疗专业人员、患者及其家属、研究人员、支付方、方案制定和宣教人员）通过共同的不懈努力，改善患者结局（即健康）、系统绩效（即医疗照护）并促进专业能力发展的过程。

多纳贝迪安作为医疗服务质量提升领域的创始人，在一次演讲中讲到：

　　"……医疗卫生保健质量是指其符合预设的优良标准的程度[8]。"

2. 设置三个级别的标准

在制定标准时，我们必须意识到标准是主观的并且存在不同视角。这点很重要。管理者可能认为医疗质量不错，但是患者和照护人员却可能认为医疗质量很差，反之亦然。再比如，许多人在接受替代或补充医疗之后认为这些是高质量医疗，但许多临床医生会认为此类医疗价值较低。

设置多个级别的标准是很有用的。19 世纪 90 年代，一本名为《追求卓越》的书风靡一时[9]，作者在书中劝勉人们力争优秀。然而，追求卓越的劝勉可能会使在困难环境下工作的人们失去动力，因为他们会认为卓越不仅是努力工作的结果，也可能是个人技巧外加良好环境的共同作用。因此，我们建议设置三个级别的标准：

- 可接受的最低标准：任何医疗服务都不得低于该标准；
- 卓越的标准：最佳医疗应达到的标准；
- 可达到的标准：例如将 75% 作为最佳医疗绩效和其余绩效分界点。

3. 通过监测临床绩效开展服务质量管理

多数监测或是源自外部的要求，或是源自内部的激励。外部要求的监测是不可避免的：卫生机构必须向上级监督机构证明医疗能力。内部激励的监

potential to drive engagement, through motivated clinical champions, close working partnerships with patients and families, and self- directed exploration of quality issues within teams and departments.

Internally motivated monitoring may be of two types:

1.troubleshooting (retrospective)

2.planned reconnaissance

a.group discussion and study (quality circles to identify, understand, propose, improve, evaluate)

b.routine surveillance (opinion surveys, performance monitoring), clinical/anecdotal (case reviews and clinical audits), as well as statistical and epidemiological on a flow of information

4: Measure wisely

One of the best books about measures is by Robert Lloyd entitled Quality Health Care: A Guide To Developing And Using Indicators (10), and his insights are discussed below.

As there are different purposes for measuring, it is as important to be clear about why you are measuring, as well as what you are measuring. In our experience, there is often a mixed agenda of learning, assurance and possibly publication uppermost in the minds of teams who are meeting to consider an improvement project.

It is crucial to have a discussion around the different purposes of measurement, and to be clear that the purpose is to measure for improvement. Lloyd (10), and the Institute for Healthcare Improvement (IHI) (11; see Table 3.1), suggest important considerations to help teams use measurement to accelerate improvement.

1. Plot data over time

2. Seek usefulness, not perfection

3. Use sampling appropriately

4. Integrate measurement into the daily routine

5. Use qualitative and quantitative data (10)

Table 3.1 Three purposes of measurement and their descriptions (11)

Aspect	Improvement	Accountability	Research
Aim	Improvement of care (efficiency and effectiveness)	Comparison, choice, reassurance, motivation for change	New knowledge (efficacy)
Methods: • Test observability	Test observable	No test, evaluate current performance	Test blinded or controlled

测则可能大大推动参与的积极性，主要可以通过以下措施：激励优秀的临床服务者，与患者及其家属建立紧密合作关系，针对团队和部门内部的质量问题开展自我分析与改进。

内部激励的监测可分为两种类型：

1．解决难题（回顾性）；

2．有计划地考核：

（1）小组讨论研究（确定、理解、提议、改进、评估的质量循环）；

（2）常规监控（意见调查和绩效监测）、临床观察／耳闻（病例回顾和临床评审）以及基于信息流的统计和流行病学调查。

4. 智慧地评估医疗质量

罗伯特·劳埃德所著的《高质量的医疗卫生保健：制定和使用评估指标的指南》[10]是有关评估医疗质量的最佳书籍之一。下面我们将讨论该作者的见解。

因为评估可以有不同目的，所以重要的是必须搞清评估的目的以及内容。根据经验，在团队开会考虑改进项目时，成员首先会想到制定包括学习、保障和发布在内的混合议程。

我们必须讨论评估的不同目的，并且明确评估是为改进而开展的。为帮助团队使用评估方法以加快服务质量的提升，劳埃德[10]和医疗卫生保健改善研究所（IHI）[11]（表 3.1）提出了以下需要考虑的要点：

1．根据时间轴绘制数据；

2．追求实用性而非尽善尽美；

3．合理利用抽样；

4．将评估与日常工作相结合；

5．定性和定量数据并用[10]。

表 3.1　三种评估目的及其描述[11]

方面	改进	责任	研究
目的	医疗保健工作的改善（效率和有效性）	改变的比较、选择、保证以及动力	新知识（效能）
方法： 检验可观察性	检验是可观察的	无检验，评估当前绩效	检验设盲或对照

continued

Aspect	Improvement	Accountability	Research
• Bias	Accept consistent bias	Measure and reduce to reduce bias	Design to eliminate bias
• Sample size	"Just enough" data, small sequential samples	Obtain 100% of available relevant data	"Just in case" data
• Flexibility of hypothesis	Flexible hypotheses, charges as learning takes place	No hypothesis	Fixed hypothesis (null hypothesis)
• Testing strategy	Sequential tests	No tests	One large test
• Determining if a change is an improvement	Run charts or Shewhart control charts (statistical process control)	No change focus (maybe compute a per cent change or rank order the results)	Hypothesis, statistical tests (t-test, F-test, chi square), p- values
• Confidentially of the data	Data used only by those involved with improvement	Data available for public consumption and review	Research subjects' indentities protected

There are also different types of information to be measured. Donabedian introduced the idea that there are three approaches to assessing quality of care–structure, process and outcome (see Figure 3.2). (2) It is important to recognise Donabedian did not intend these to be 'attributes of quality', they are simply types of information, and provide a useful framework to help in structuring the measures and other information to be gathered in any project.

STRUCTURE
(Including personnel, equipment, buildings, record systems, finance, supplies and facilities)

PROCESS
(Incorporating all aspects of the performance, technical and interpersonal, of activities of care)

OUTCOME
(The results of care/service)

Figure 3.2　Donabedian's 'structure, process, outcome' (12)

■ An overview of the models of quality improvement

Programmes of quality improvement originated in industry: within that sector, these methodologies have been responsible for driving increased productivity, efficiency and client and employee satisfaction.

续表

方面	改进	责任	研究
• 偏倚	接受一致性偏倚	测量并减少偏倚	进行设计以消除偏倚
• 样本量	"正好足够"的数据，少量连续样本	获得 100% 可用的相关数据	"以备不时之需"的数据
• 假设灵活性	灵活的假设，随着学习的深入而变化	无假设	固定假设（无效假设）
• 检验策略	序贯检验	无检验	一项大型检验
• 确定某一变化是否带来服务质量的改进	运作质量管理图表或 Shewhart 控制图（统计过程控制）	无变化重点（可计算变化的百分数或对结果排序）	假设、统计检验（t 检验，F 检验，卡方）、p 值
• 数据保密	仅允许参与改进的人员使用数据	可供公众使用和查阅的数据	研究对象的身份受到保护

　　需要评估的信息也有不同类型。多纳贝迪安介绍了评估医疗卫生服务质量的三个维度：结构、过程和结果（图 3.2）[2]。值得注意的是，多纳贝迪安并未将这三个维度视为"质量的属性"，这些只是信息类型，可作为框架来帮助归类项目中收集的评估数据和其他信息。

结构
（包括人员、设备、建筑、记录系统、财务、耗材和设施）

过程
（把医疗服务活动相关的各方面的绩效、技术和人际关系进行结合）

结果
（即医疗保健/服务的结果）

图 3.2　多纳贝迪安的"结构 – 过程 – 结果"模型[12]

■ **质量改善模型概述**

　　质量改善项目起源于工业界：在业内，这些方法论一直在推动提高生产率、效率以及客户和员工满意度。

Since the early 1990s, healthcare organisations have adopted these approaches and have driven through improvement and reform projects, such as streamlining the process of referral from primary to secondary care, and introducing evidenced-based bundles of care into critical care. The approaches taken include:

- *Total Quality Management (TQM)*
- *Continuous Quality Improvement (CQI)*
- *Business Process Reengineering (BPR)*
- *Rapid Cycle Change*
- *Lean Thinking*
- *Six Sigma*

A full explanation of these models is available in the excellent review of quality improvement models by Powell et al. (13)

Powell and colleagues highlight that it is important to realise there is no single right methodology to use in quality improvement; to date, there is no evidence to suggest that one model is more effective than others.

Of greater interest is the finding that the different models of quality improvement all use similar implementation approaches. Successful implementation depends on the presence of 'necessary conditions'. Ensuring the following conditions are in place is crucial to the task of population healthcare improvement:

- *provision of practical and human resources to enable quality improvement (train and build both capacity and capability)*
- *the active engagement of health professionals, especially doctors (consider and work with the incentives – both intrinsic and extrinsic)*
- *sustained managerial focus and attention*
- *the use of multifaceted interventions*
- *coordinated action at all levels of the healthcare system (particularly relevant in a population-based initiative)*
- *substantial investment in training and development*
- *the availability of robust and timely data through supported IT systems*

It can be argued that the context in which interventions are embedded is more important than the model used.

■ Quality improvement – 'a contact sport'

The phrase 'patient safety and quality improvement is a contact sport' highlights that the existing interdependencies among professional groups, management, academia and patients demand concerted collaborative effort across interdependent themes and work. It is not easy.

自 1990 年代初以来，医疗保健机构引入了这些方法，并借此推动了改进和改革项目，例如：简化初级到二级医疗的转诊流程，以及将循证医疗引入重症监护。具体采取的方法包括：

- 全面质量管理（TQM）；
- 持续性质量改善（CQI）；
- 业务流程再造（BPR）；
- 快速周期变化；
- 精益思维；
- 六西格玛。

鲍威尔等人[13]对这些质量改善模型进行了绝佳综述并对各模型进行了全面解析。

鲍威尔及其同事强调，质量改善没有唯一的正确方法；迄今为止，没有证据表明一种模型比其他模型更有效。

更值得关注的一点是，不同的质量改善模型在实施时颇为相似。实施成功与否取决于我们是否具备"必要条件"。要想人群的医疗保健改进获得成功，我们必须确保以下几个条件：

- 提供医疗实践和人力资源以改善医疗质量（培训并建立相应能力与资源）；
- 医疗专业人员，特别是医生的积极参与（考虑并采用内在和外在的激励措施）；
- 管理重点的持续化和受到关注；
- 采用多方面的干预措施；
- 在医疗卫生保健体系各个层面采取协调一致的行动（特别是在基于人群的倡议中）；
- 持续投资专业能力的培训发展；
- 通过 IT 系统的支持以获得稳定及时的数据。

可以认为：干预措施所在的环境要比使用的模型更为重要。

■ 改善医疗质量——一项"接触性运动"

"改善患者安全和医疗质量是一种接触性运动"这句话是要强调：专业医疗团队、管理层、学术界和患者之间需要共同努力，跨越彼此独立的工作主题和工作内容。这绝非易事。

It helps to have clear ideas about the deliverables from the quality improvement process. Batalden and Davidoff (7) provide a good starting point regarding the domains of interest in quality improvement:

1. Healthcare processes within systems
2. Variation and measurement
3. Leading, following and making changes in healthcare
4. Collaboration
5. Social context and accountability
6. Developing new, locally useful knowledge

These authors highlight that the definition of healthcare improvement arises from the conviction that healthcare will not meet its full potential until change-making becomes a routine part of everyone's job, in all parts of the healthcare system. (7)

The culture in healthcare delivery is steeped in historical professional and disciplinary silos. Even within professional groups, the lack of joined-up, consistent working can negatively affect the quality of care provided, and staff morale.

To achieve dissemination of the changes and sustainable improvement across populations, there is a need for considerable capacity-building, together with relentless and unwavering attention from senior leaders.

To address Continuous Quality Improvement at a population level, a five-stage plan for improvement is required (Display 3.1).

Display 3.1 A five-stage plan for improvement

Systems and resources	Performance monitoring and adjustment
1. Plan for continuous change	2. Understand the process
	3. Eliminate errors
	4. Remove the slack
	5. Reduce variation

■ Questions for reflection
  • *What do you think are the dimensions or domains of quality in healthcare*
  • *Can you describe at least one example of a quality issue in relation to each domain from a personal as well as a patient perspective?*

这有助于我们清楚地认识到质量改善过程可取得哪些切实成果。关于质量改善的领域，巴塔尔登和大卫杜夫[7]提供了一个很好的起点：

1. 医疗卫生保健体系内的流程；

2. 变量和测量；

3. 医疗卫生保健中的领导、跟进和改变；

4. 协作；

5. 社会背景和责任；

6. 开发新的、对当地有用的知识。

作者们强调，医疗保健质量改善的定义自这样一种信念中产生：医疗保健系统只有在改变成为每人工作的常态时才能够发挥其全部潜力[7]。

医疗卫生保健供给文化深受专业历史和学科领域影响。即使在专科医疗团体内部，如果缺乏合作沟通，持续性工作也会在所提供的医疗护理质量和员工职业操守方面产生负面影响。

为了在人群中传播变化，实现持续性改善，我们需要开展大规模的能力建设，同时需要高层领导持续不懈地关注改进过程。

为了解决群体层面的持续性质量改善（CQI），需制定一个包含五个阶段的改进计划（场景 3.1）。

场景 3.1　五阶段的改进计划

系统和资源	绩效监测和调整
1. 为连续变化制定计划	2. 了解流程
	3. 消除错误
	4. 杜绝懈怠
	5. 减少偏差

■ 思考题

- 您认为医疗卫生服务质量包含哪些方面或领域？

- 您能否从个人和患者的角度描述上述领域存在的质量问题（每个领域至少举一例）？

- *What can you do to encourage monitoring as part of your quality improvement commitment?*
- *In what ways is it possible to harness the power of staff and patient narratives?*
- *What is the concept of 'building will' for change, and what are the possible benefits of patient and staff narratives?*
- *How do the domains of quality draw on different skill sets, and what are the implications for your future career aspirations?*

References

(1) National Advisory Group on the Safety of Patients in England. A promise to learn – a commitment to act. Improving the safety of patients in England. [London]: Department of Health; 2013: 4.

(2) Donabedian A. An introduction to quality assurance in health care. New York: Oxford University Press; 2003.

(3) Donabedian A. An introduction to quality assurance in health care. New York: Oxford University Press; 2003: xi-xii.

(4) Donabedian A. An introduction to quality assurance in health care. New York: Oxford University Press; 2003: xxiii.

(5) Institute of Medicine. Medicare: a strategy for quality assurance, Volume 1. Washington, DC: National Academies Press; 1990: 21.

(6) Institute of Medicine. Crossing the quality chasm: a new health system for the 21st century. Washington, DC: National Academies Press; 2001.

(7) Batalden PB, Davidoff F. What is quality improvement and how can it transform healthcare? Qual Saf Health Care. 2007; 16(1): 2-3.

- 在质量改善中，您可以采取什么措施推动绩效监测？

- 如何利用工作人员和患者讲述的案例评估服务质量？

- 如何理解医疗机构内的参与者为质量改善而树立意愿？利用工作人员和患者讲述的故事或案例可发挥什么作用？

- 不同质量领域如何影响不同技能组合？对您未来的职业抱负有什么影响？

参 考 文 献

(8) Gray M. Muir Gray: Setting standards for systems of care. The BMJ [Blog]. 2012 Nov 15. Available from: http://blogs.bmj.com/bmj/2012/11/15/muir-gray-setting-standards-for-systems-of-care/

(9) Peters TJ. In search of excellence: lessons from America's best run companies. New York: Harper & Row; 1991.

(10) Lloyd RC. Quality health care: a guide to developing and using indicators. Sudbury, Mass.: Jones and Bartlett; 2004.

(11) Solberg L, Mosser G, McDonald S. The three faces of performance improvement: improvement, accountability and research. Joint Commission Journal on Quality Improvement. Mar 1997; 23: 135-147.

(12) Whiteley S, Ellis R, Broomfield S. Health and social care management. Sevenoaks: Edward Arnold; 1996.

(13) Powell AE, Rushmer RK, Davies HTO. A systematic narrative review of quality improvement models in healthcare. [Dundee]: Social Dimensions of Health Institute, Universities of Dundee and St. Andrews; 2008.

3.3 Managing knowledge that serves populations

As knowledge management is the subject of Book 4 in our Healthcare Transformation series, we offer only a brief introduction here and encourage you to read Knowledge Management.

■ Healthcare is a knowledge business

It is clear that healthcare is in the business of improving health, although some people think of healthcare as in the business of real estate, and some think of it as in the business of technology, such as scanners, drugs and sterilising equipment. By contrast, healthcare is a perfect example of a knowledge business.

Although chief executives of hospitals must manage the real estate, they employ 'knowledge' workers, that is, people who add value because they know more about a particular topic than anyone else in the population. It is knowledge that creates the technology, and knowledge that determines when it should be used for best value.

In most health services, knowledge is managed much less carefully than money or buildings. In health services around the world, it is relatively easy to discover the names of property or building managers, but not the names of knowledge managers. Indeed, in many healthcare organisations, no-one holds this responsibility.

■ Knowledge management responsibilities in population medicine

Knowledge is critically important in achieving good outcomes for patients and in maximising value from clinical services. Therefore, clinicians with managerial responsibilities (whole- or part-time) should include a responsibility for managing knowledge in their brief, and assume this responsibility even if it has not been given to them. Furthermore, as knowledge is shared and exchanged in populations, such clinicians should take responsibility for the management of knowledge for the whole population in need, not just for those patients in contact with the service.

The management of knowledge for the population is one of the key responsibilities and new skills of population medicine, partly because any service is in competition with other providers. The traditional responsibility towards knowledge management is that all professionals who work within the specialist service should be up to date with best current evidence. This type of responsibility, however, is focused on self-improvement for a limited number of individuals and could have potentially negative consequences for the care of the

第 3 节　为各种人群服务的知识管理

知识管理是"医疗卫生保健转型"<u>丛书</u>第四册的主题，在此仅作简要介绍，建议阅读第四册《知识管理》的相关主题。

■ 医疗保健是知识型行业

很明显，医疗卫生保健是一个改善健康的行业；尽管有人认为它是不动产行业，也有人将其视为技术型行业，如扫描仪、药物和消毒设备。但相比来说，医疗卫生保健是知识型行业的完美范例。

虽然首席执行官必须管理医院，但他们聘用的是知识型工作者，是比其他人更了解特定知识而为医院带来价值的人。知识创造了技术，知识决定了技术的最佳使用时机。

在大多数医疗服务中，管理知识的仔细程度远逊于管理资金或建筑物。在世界各地的医疗卫生保健机构中，找到资产或建筑物管理者的姓名相对容易，但找到知识管理者的姓名很难。实际上，在许多医疗保健组织中，没有人承担这项职责。

■ 群医学中知识管理的职责

知识是临床诊疗中为患者带来良好结局和最大价值极为重要的部分。因此，即使承担着管理职责的临床医生（无论全职或兼职）没有被赋予知识管理的职责，也应在其工作简报中包括这项任务。此外，知识是在人群中交流共享的，上述临床医生不仅应为求医患者进行知识管理，还应为有需求的全体人群负责。

人群知识管理是群医学的一项关键职责和全新技能，部分原因是任何服务都在与其他提供者竞争。知识管理的传统职责是，在专科工作的所有专业人员都应该不停地更新最新的证据。但是，由于此类职责仅聚焦于少数人的自我完善，可能会给接受医疗的人群带来潜在不良结果。在这种情况下，现

population served. In this situation, it is not clear who has overall responsibility for meeting the information needs of the wider community of clinicians serving the population in need (see Display 3.2). Part of the reason for a lack of clarity about who is responsible for managing knowledge for the population in need is that certain specific responsibilities for information provision may rest with different healthcare professionals.

The roles and responsibilities of three types of clinician in relation to knowledge provision are shown in Table 3.2; however, each role needs to be developed and the coordination among them improved.

Display 3.2 A population-based clinical practice simulation

Scenario: You are a clinician with responsibility for orthopaedic and rheumatology services for a population of 500,000 people

Who is responsible for ensuring that:
• a new general practitioner in the population served knows the referral criteria for back pain?
• patients are assured that the service provided in their locality serves them better than the service in the neighbouring locality?
• the hip re-operation rate in your locality is within an acceptable range?
• older people in the population know about fragility fractures and how they can be prevented?
• pharmacists and general practitioners know the best-value drug treatment for rheumatoid arthritis?
• people who make decisions about licensing alcohol understand what they can do to prevent trauma?
• patients considering knee replacement understand the probability and nature of the risks of the operation as well as they understand the benefits?
• when surgeons retire, the key lessons they have learnt are captured and passed on?

Table 3.2 Roles and responsibilities for knowledge provision for three groups of healthcare professionals

Healthcare professional and their responsibility to knowledge provision	Action required
General practitioners (GPs) have a clear responsibility to ensure that: • they have access to best current knowledge • the patients who attend for consultations receive the knowledge they need	In a health centre at which there is a team of GPs and other clinicians, one clinician should take lead responsibility and adopt the role of chief knowledge officer
Specialist clinicians working in hospitals or mental health services have an important part to play in ensuring that all patients directly supported by the service receive information about their condition, and the probability of the benefit and the harm relating to the different treatment options for their condition	Clinicians who are medical managers of a service should consider the knowledge needs of: • staff in the specialist service • GPs, particularly those new to the locality • pharmacists in private community pharmacies • physiotherapists in the community service and private practice • patients who reach the service

在还不清楚到底应该由谁来满足广大临床医生团体的信息需求（场景 3.2）；此事尚不明晰的部分原因是：提供信息的特定职责可能分属于不同的医疗卫生保健人员。

表 3.2 列出了三类临床医生在提供知识方面的角色和职责。每个角色都需要发展，并且需要增进彼此之间的协调。

场景 3.2　以人群为基础的临床实践模拟

情况：您是一名临床医生，负责为 50 万人提供骨科疾病和风湿病服务。

你要为下列问题负责：

- 新全科医生知道他所服务的人群中的腰痛转诊标准吗？
- 与周边地区相比，患者是否知道当地为他们提供了更好的医疗吗？
- 所在地区的髋关节再手术率是否在可接受的范围内？
- 人群中的老年人了解脆性骨折以及如何预防吗？
- 药剂师和全科医生了解类风湿关节炎最佳药物治疗措施吗？
- 考虑做膝关节置换的患者了解手术风险、性质以及好处吗？
- 批准酒精类销售许可证的决策者知道采取什么措施来预防创伤吗？
- 外科医生在退休时，他们学到的主要经验教训会被保留并传承下去吗？

表 3.2　三组医疗卫生保健专业人员在提供知识方面的角色和职责

医疗卫生专业人员及知识提供职责	需要采取的行动
全科医生有一项明确的职责，即确保： - 自己能够获得最好最新的知识； - 就医患者能获得所需的知识	在由全科医生和其他临床医生组成的医疗中心，由一名临床医生承担主要责任并担任首席知识官
在医院或精神卫生医疗机构工作的专科医生有一个重要角色，即确保该服务部门直接支持的所有患者都获得有关自己病情的信息以及不同治疗方案可能带来的损益概率	医疗机构管理岗的临床医生应考虑以下人员的知识需求： - 从事专科医疗的员工； - 全科医生，特别是本地新来的全科医生； - 社区私人药房的药剂师； - 在社区服务和私人执业中的物理治疗师； - 寻求医疗服务的患者

continued

Healthcare professional and their responsibility to knowledge provision	Action required
Directors of public health (DsPH) have a responsibility for delivering public health services to a defined population. Just as it is a public health responsibility to ensure that the population has clean clear water, should it not be a responsibility for the public health service to ensure clean clear knowledge? (1)	Directors of public health must ensure that everyone in the local population (including people who do not have a GP) receives the knowledge they need, particularly knowledge relating to how to stay healthy and prevent disease

■ Knowledge as a driver for better value healthcare

The three drivers of what Manual Castells has described as the third era of industrial revolution are knowledge, the Internet and citizens. (2) These drivers are also highly relevant to healthcare, and in particular to population medicine.

It is not common for a clinician to face competition when designing and creating systems and networks for a population. By contrast, when trying to ensure that all professionals and patients within a population receive unbiased, clearly presented, up-to-date knowledge, the clinician practising population medicine faces intense competition from the media, particularly the Internet.

Key features of the sources of competition to unbiased information about healthcare include:

- *multiple sources of knowledge*
- *no control over what can be found through some knowledge sources, such as the Internet and newspapers*
- *no editorial control of content of some knowledge sources, for example, the Internet*
- *lack of an evidence base, for example, newspaper campaigns about screening for prostate cancer in which celebrities are used as figureheads*
- *easy access to knowledge sources, for example, many patients access the Internet both before and after a consultation*
- *lack of disclosure by patients to clinicians about accessing other knowledge sources for fear of upsetting the clinician or of being reprimanded*

It is therefore necessary for those who pay for or manage healthcare resources to compete with other sources of knowledge in the knowledge 'marketplace', particularly the Internet.

■ Classifying knowledge

Knowledge is classified as either generalisable (relevant everywhere) or particular (relevant only to a particular patient or service). Generalisable knowledge can be further classified into several categories (see Figure 3.3).

续表

医疗卫生专业人员及知识提供职责	需要采取的行动
公共卫生部门主任负责为特定人群提供公共卫生服务。正如确保人群拥有干净清洁的水是公共卫生的一项职责，确保获得清晰明确的知识难道不也应该是公共卫生职责之一吗？[1]	公共卫生主任必须确保当地人群中的每个人（包括未与全科医生签约的人）均能够获得所需的知识，尤其是如何保持健康和预防疾病方面的知识

■ 知识是提高医疗卫生保健价值的驱动力

曼纽尔·卡斯特描述了第三次工业革命时代的 3 个驱动因素：知识、互联网和民众[2]。这些驱动因素也与医疗保健，特别是群医学，高度相关。

在为人群设计和创建相关系统和网络时，临床医生很少遇到竞争。相反，当试图确保人群中所有专业人员和患者获取客观公正、清晰表述、及时更新的知识时，从事群医学的临床医生要面临着来自媒体，尤其是互联网的激烈竞争。对于客观公正的医疗卫生保健信息，其竞争来源的主要特征包括：

- 多种知识来源。
- 无法控制人群从互联网和报纸等知识来源获取什么样的内容。
- 无法对互联网等知识来源的内容进行编辑管控。
- 缺少证据基础，如报纸利用名人炒作前列腺癌筛查活动。
- 容易获取知识的来源，如许多患者在就医前后访问互联网。
- 患者不向临床医生透露访问其他知识来源的信息，因为他们担心引起临床医生反感或受到谴责。

因此，对于购买或管理医疗卫生保健资源的人来说，有必要与知识"市场"中的其他知识来源相竞争，尤其是互联网。

■ 知识分类

知识可分为通识（处处相关）或专识（仅与特定患者或医疗照护相关）。通识可进一步分为以下几类（图 3.3）。

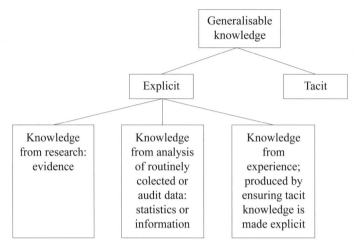

Figure 3.3   Three types of explicit knowledge

■ Managing different types of knowledge

The management of knowledge involves not only its creation but also its use, both of which require good management. In health services, the management of all types of generalisable knowledge needs to be improved.

Improving the management of knowledge from experience

> *Tacit knowledge consists partly of technical skills – the kind of informal, hard-to-pin down skills captured in the term 'know- how'. A master craftsman after years of experience develops a wealth of expertise 'at his finger-tips'. But he is often unable to articulate the scientific or technical principles behind what he knows.*

> *At the same time, tacit knowledge has an important cognitive dimension. It consists of mental models, beliefs, and perspectives so ingrained that we take them for granted, and therefore cannot easily articulate them. (3)*

Knowledge from the experience of professionals

Of the three types of explicit knowledge, knowledge from experience is the type least well managed. It needs to be created by converting tacit knowledge into explicit forms, for example, by:

- *interviewing staff as they leave (exit interviews or knowledge harvesting) to find out what their successor needs to know and how the service could change for the better*

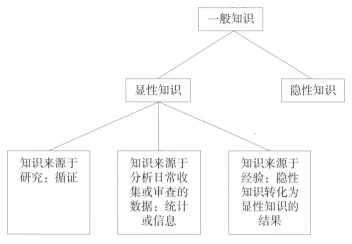

图 3.3　三种显性知识

■ 管理不同类型的知识

知识管理不仅包括创造，还包括应用，而两者均需要良好的管理。在医疗卫生保健中，所有类型的通识管理都需要提高。

改善来源于经验的知识管理

隐性知识包括技术技能——一种非正式的、难以确定的技能，即所谓的"诀窍"。有多年经验的熟练工匠具有丰富的专业知识，"唯手熟尔"，但通常他无法阐述其背后的科学或技术原理。

同时，隐性知识具有重要的认知维度，它由思维模式、信念和观点组成。这些认知往往根深蒂固，以至于我们将其视为理所当然而无法轻易表达出来[3]。

来自专业人员经验的知识

在三类显性知识中，来自经验的知识是最不好管理的类型。以下方式可以将隐性知识转化为显性知识：

• 对离职员工进行访谈（离职采访或知识收集），了解其继任者所需的知识和如何将服务变得更好。

- *celebrating successes and profiting from failures, by ensuring that there is time for reflection and discussion after a project is finished*
- *building a casebook in which people record the outcomes of projects, successful and unsuccessful, and the lessons learned*
- *developing partnerships with other services and arranging exchanges so that members of staff can experience different approaches to the same job in different contexts*
- *using the Map of Medicine® and other software for care pathways to make tacit knowledge explicit in a graphic medium, which is much more accessible for the majority of people*

In addition to these formal techniques of converting tacit to explicit knowledge, learning can be garnered during informal situations. The clinician leading a service needs to create a culture in which discussing the service in a social setting is seen as valuable. The cultural change required is one best described as the transformation to a learning organisation.

> *Peter Senge, who popularized learning organizations in his book The Fifth Discipline, described them as places 'where people continually expand their capacity to create the results they truly desire, where new and expansive patterns of thinking are nurtured, where collective aspiration is set free, and where people are continually learning how to learn together'. (4)*

Knowledge from the experience of patients

The importance of harnessing the knowledge of patients, not only for the purposes of learning but also as part of developing an emotional bond with patients, has been emphasised elsewhere (see section 1.3).

Improving the management of knowledge from data

Hitherto, the information used by managers has been restricted to finance and activity data. In the 21st century, the priority will be to manage services using information about quality and outcome. Information on quality can be collected through audits undertaken in the institution in which the medical manager works. To obtain information on outcomes, which is essential for the assessment of value, data inputs from the whole system of care are required.

For instance, to gain information about the outcome of hip replacement, data are required about:

- *the pre-operative health status of the individual*
- *the individual's health status three months after the hip has been replaced, long after the patient has left hospital*

Thus, obtaining information about outcomes, including clinical measures and patient-reported outcome measures, requires the cooperation of the entire network of services providing care for the population, and of individual patients seen by the service.

- 庆祝成功，吸取失败教训，确保在项目完成后有时间进行反思和讨论。
- 编写案例集，记录成功和失败的项目结果，以及所获经验教训。
- 与其他医疗机构发展伙伴关系并安排交流活动，使工作人员体验到不同背景下相同工作的不同做法。
- 使用医学地图（Map of Medicine®）或医疗路径的其他软件，通过图形媒介使隐性知识变得清晰，便于大多数人学习。

除了上述将隐性知识转化为显性知识的正规方式外，也可在非正式情况下获得知识。临床医生作为医疗机构的领导者，需要创造一种文化，在这种文化中，在社交场合下讨论医疗服务被视为有价值的。转变为学习型组织是对这种文化所需变化的最好诠释。

> 彼得·圣吉在其《第五项修炼》中推广了学习型组织，将此类机构描述为"在这里，人们不断扩展能力以创造自己真正想要结果；在这里，全新广阔的思维模式被培育；在这里，集体意愿被释放出来；在这里，人们不断学习如何共同学习"[4]。

来自患者体验的知识

第 1 章第 3 节强调了利用患者知识的重要性，这不仅是为了学习的目的，也是与患者建立情感纽带的一部分。

改善数据来源的知识管理

迄今为止，管理者使用的信息仅局限于财务和活动数据。在 21 世纪，首要任务将是使用有关质量和结局的信息来管理医疗服务。质量信息可通过评估医疗管理者的机构来收集。为了获取对价值评估至关重要的结果信息，需要输入来自整个医疗系统中的数据。例如，为了获得髋关节置换手术结局的信息，则需要以下数据：

- 患者术前健康状况。
- 髋关节置换 3 个月后以及出院更久后的健康状况。

因此，要获得包括临床评估和患者报告的结局评估在内的有关结局的信息，就需要为人群提供医疗照护的整个网络体系以及接受医疗的个体患者之间的合作。

The debate about the relative importance of process and outcome measures has attracted much attention. There is now a consensus that, although both are necessary, in future people who manage healthcare will be held to account not only for the quality and safety of the care they provide to patients but also for the value derived from the resources. There are two ways in which to estimate value by:

1.relating outcome to expenditure

2.comparing services, and plotting the position of each service on the value map shown in Figure 3.4

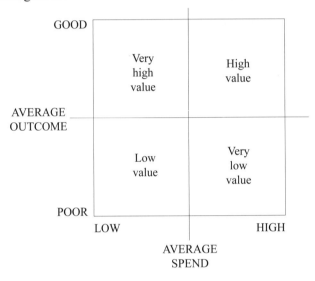

Figure 3.4   The value matrix

It is vital to assess effectiveness in relation to expenditure; indeed, it could be considered negligent not to do so. Even quality improvement, the target of the last decade, needs to be assessed in relation to the cost of achieving any change in the level of performance. Bob Brook, one of the creators of the quality movement, signalled the end of the quality improvement era in 2010 when he published an article subtitled 'Long Live Increasing Value'. (5) The measurement of quality is the means by which institutions can be held to account. The assessment of value, however, requires knowledge to be related to populations and not to institutions.

Improving the management of population-based and not just institution-based knowledge

The principle of population accountability was first developed by Mark Friedman. (6) Friedman identified the overlap of, but difference between, outcomes for 'populations' and outcomes for 'customers and communities'. Although Friedman's focus is education, his analysis is relevant to healthcare, especially the relationship between population and performance accountability, which can be directly transferred into a healthcare setting (see Table 3.3).

关于过程和结局评估孰轻孰重的争论由来已久。虽然两者都实属必要：但现已达成共识，未来，医疗卫生管理者不仅为患者的医疗服务质量和安全性负责，还要为从资源中获取的价值负责。可以通过以下两种方式评估价值。

1. 将结局和支出挂钩。

2. 比较各种医疗服务，在价值图上绘制每种医疗卫生服务的位置（图 3.4）。

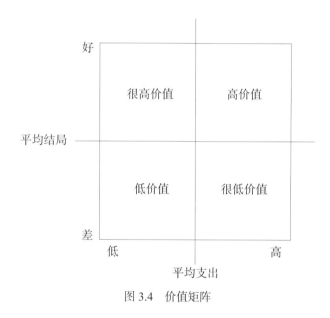

图 3.4 价值矩阵

评估与支出相关的效果是很重要的；实际上，不做评估可视为工作的疏漏。即使改善质量（过去 10 年的工作目标）也需要在绩效层面评估取得成效的成本。

质量运动的创建者之一鲍勃·布鲁克在 2010 年发表了一篇《增加价值万岁》的文章，标志着改善质量时代的结束[5]。评估质量是使医疗机构承担责任的手段，然而评估价值则需要与人群而非医疗机构相关的知识。

改善以人群为基础而不仅仅是以机构为基础的知识管理

马克·弗里德曼最早提出了人群责任制的原理[6]。弗里德曼确定了"人群"的结果与"客户和社区"的结果之间彼此重叠，但有所差异。尽管弗里德曼的重点是在教育方面，但他的分析与医疗保健也相关，尤其是可以直接把人群与绩效责任之间的关系转移到医疗卫生保健机构中（表 3.3）。

Table 3.3 The relationship between population and performance accountability

The seven population accountability questions	The seven performance accountability questions
• What are the quality of life conditions we want for our children, adults and families who live in our community? • What would those conditions look like if we could see them? • How can we measure those conditions? • How are we doing on the most important of these measures? • Who are the partners that have a role to play in doing better? • What works to do better, including no- cost and low-cost ideas? • What do we propose to do?	• Who are our customers? • How can we measure if our customers are better off? • How can we measure if we are delivering services well? • How are we doing on the most important of these measures? • Who are the partners that have a role to play in doing better? • What works to do better, including no-cost and low- cost ideas? • What do we propose to do?

In an era of resource constraint, it is important to create what has been called 'public value for the population' (7) in addition to providing value for individual patients using the service. The creation of value is critical in a context of increasing demands for transparency from both Government and civil society.

■ The need for a chief knowledge officer

As knowledge is an important resource in any public health organisation, it should be an important contributor in our pursuit of 'population health', 'patient experience', and 'value'. And as with the management of other important resources, the management of knowledge requires leadership, and a senior member of staff should be given overall responsibility for managing it. This responsibility can be encapsulated within the role of a chief knowledge officer (8), which was first developed by the private sector in the USA. It is important to emphasise that the chief knowledge officer is a leadership role, not a job. A member of the senior management team, preferably a person directly accountable to the chief executive, should be given the responsibility for ensuring that knowledge created and used by an organisation is well managed. If knowledge in the organisation is not well managed, the chief knowledge officer should be given a budget and the authority to mobilise resources to rectify the situation.

表 3.3　人群与绩效责任制之间的关系

7 个人群责任制的问题	7 个绩效责任制的问题
• 我们希望为住在社区中的儿童、成人以及家庭提供什么质量的生活条件？ • 如果我们能看到这些条件时，它们是什么样呢？ • 我们如何评估这些条件？ • 我们对评估工作中最重要的方面做得如何？ • 谁是我们改善工作的伙伴？ • 哪些方法可以做得更好？包括无成本和低成本方法。 • 我们应该做什么？	• 我们的客户是谁？ • 对那些客户境况较好，我们该如何评估呢？ • 当我们能很好地提供服务时，我们该如何评估？ • 我们在评估工作中最重要的方面做得如何？ • 当我们想把工作做得更好时，谁是我们的合作伙伴？ • 哪些方法可以做得更好？包括无成本和低成本的方法。 • 我们应该做什么？

在资源匮乏的年代，除了接受医疗的个体患者提供价值外，重要的是要创造所谓的"公众价值"[7]。在政府和社会对透明度要求越来越高的背景下，创造价值至关重要。

■ 对首席知识官的要求

知识是任何公共卫生组织的重要资源，因此也应是我们所追求的"人群健康""患者体验"和"价值"的重要贡献者。与其他重要资源的管理一样，知识管理也需要具有领导力并由一位高级职员全权负责管理。首席知识官的角色中包括这类职责[8]。这个职位最初由美国私营部门设置。值得强调的是，首席知识官是一种领导角色，而非一项工作。一名高级管理团队的成员——直接对首席执行官负责——可被赋予职权来管理机构创造和使用的知识。如果组织中的知识管理不善，管理团队应给首席知识官预算和授权来调用资源纠正这种情况。

In a healthcare setting, the medical director is usually the person best qualified to be given the role and responsibility of chief knowledge officer. In turn, the chief knowledge officer can ask each clinical director to take on the corresponding role and responsibility for the relevant directorates. Although it is possible to combine the role and responsibility of a chief knowledge officer with those of a chief information officer, the latter post is usually restricted to the management of data and the production of financial and activity information for management. The typical responsibilities of a chief knowledge officer in a healthcare setting are shown in Box 3.1.

Box 3.1 Responsibilities of a chief knowledge officer in a healthcare setting

• Capturing the tacit knowledge within and about the service and making sure it is used
• Identifying and procuring the sources of evidence that the service requires
• Ensuring that all information for patients is unbiased and clear
• Developing the annual reports for clinical systems and services
• Identifying the wider community of professionals caring for the population served by the service and ensuring their knowledge needs are ascertained and met
• Ensuring the board and senior management team base their decisions on best current evidence

The aim of a chief knowledge officer is to get knowledge into action, an activity increasingly characterised as knowledge translation, defined by the Canadian Institute of Health Research as:

... a dynamic and iterative process that includes synthesis, dissemination, exchange and ethically sound application of knowledge. (9)

In an era when financial resources are constrained, the infinite resource that is knowledge can increase value for the population and for individual patients. (10)

The British Standards Institution (BSI) has produced a Guide to Good Practice in Knowledge Management (11), in which are identified the qualities that a chief knowledge officer might need (see Box 3.2).

Box 3.2 Qualities for a chief knowledge officer

• A 'frontline' background

• The ability to command the respect of senior management

• A deep understanding of the organisation's business and culture

• A high level of technological literacy

• A tolerance of ambiguity and the ability to work with minimal structure

在医疗机构中，医务主任通常是最有资格担任首席知识官角色和职责的人。反之，首席知识官可以要求每位临床主任在其所管辖的部门中承担相应的角色和责任。尽管可将首席知识官和首席信息官的角色和责任结合起来，但后者岗位通常仅限于数据、财务成果和活动信息的管理。专栏 3.1 列出了首席知识官在医疗机构中的典型职责。

专栏 3.1　首席知识官在医疗机构中的职责

- 获取医疗服务内部和相关的隐性知识并确保其使用。
- 识别并获得医疗服务所需的证据来源。
- 确保为患者提供的所有信息公正客观且清晰。
- 编制临床系统和医疗服务的年度报告。
- 确定专业人员所服务的更为广泛的人群范围，并确保识别和满足他们的知识需求。
- 确保董事会和高级管理团队的决策是建立在现有最佳证据之上的。

首席知识官的目标是将知识付诸行动，这种活动越来越有知识翻译的特征，加拿大卫生研究院将其定义为：

> ……一个动态且迭代的过程，在应用时，应包括知识的综合、传播、交流和合乎伦理的应用[9]。

在经济资源匮乏的时代，知识作为无限资源，可为人群和个体患者增加价值[10]。

英国标准协会（BSI）编写了《知识管理的良好实践指南》，其中确定了首席知识官可能需要的素质（专栏 3.2）。

专栏 3.2　首席知识官的素质

- 具有"临床一线"背景；
- 有能力得到高层管理人员的尊重；
- 对组织的事业和文化有深刻的了解；
- 高水平的技术素养；
- 能够容忍模棱两可，并有能力与最简结构的团队开展工作。

Directors of public health as chief knowledge officers for health knowledge

On 28 July 2010, through Resolution 64/292, the United Nations General Assembly recognised the human right to water and sanitation, and acknowledged that clean drinking water and sanitation are essential to the realisation of all human rights. (12) Knowledge is like water. Everyone has a need for and a right to clean clear knowledge, in the same way that they have a need for and a right to clean clear water.

Ignorance is like cholera, a water-borne disease. It cannot be managed by any one individual; it requires the organised efforts of society. Thus, it is a public health responsibility. The responsibility for ensuring that everyone in the population – professionals, patients and the public – has access to clean clear knowledge could be added to the existing responsibilities of directors of public health. This new responsibility could be discharged through the traditional public health method of needs assessment: by identifying groups whose needs for knowledge are not being adequately met and then through the performance management of healthcare organisations with the main responsibility for delivering knowledge to clinicians and patients who have reached the organisations' services.

In addition, to ensure that clean clear knowledge is available everywhere, directors of public health could work with:

- *the public library service*
- *social services*
- *the third sector of voluntary and community organisations*

■ Questions for reflection

- *If you were given the responsibility of being chief knowledge officer and the necessary authority, what would be your first three actions?*
- *How could better use be made of the Internet as a means of managing knowledge for a population?*

References

(1) Pang T et al. A 15th Grand Challenge for Global Public Health. Lancet. 2006; 367: 284–286.

(2) Castells M. The Network Society. Oxford: Blackwell; 2009.

(3) Nonaka I. (1991) The Knowledge-Creating Company. Harvard Business Review. 1991; 69(6): 14–15.

(4) Harvard Business Review. On Knowledge Management. Boston: Harvard Business School Press. 1987; 49.

(5) Brook RH. The End of the Quality Improvement Movement. JAMA. 2010; 304: 1831–1832.

(6) Friedman M. Trying Hard is not Good Enough: how to produce measurable improvements for both customers and communities. Indiana: Trafford; 2005.

作为首席知识官的公共卫生主任应具有的医疗卫生知识

2010 年 7 月 28 日，联合国大会通过第 64/292 号决议，承认清洁饮用水和卫生设施对于实现人权至关重要 [12]。知识就像水。每个人都离不开它，而且有权利得到清晰明确的知识。正如每个人也需要并有权得到清洁和干净的水。

无知就像霍乱，是一种经"水"传播的疾病。它不能由任何个体管理；而需要社会有组织的努力。因此，这是一项公共卫生责任，确保人群中的每一个人（专业人员、患者和公众）均可以获取清晰明确的知识，并将这一责任纳入公共卫生主任现有的职责中。可以通过传统的对公共卫生需求进行评估方法来履行这一新的职责：通过确定哪些人还未充分满足其知识需求，解决的办法可以是用医疗卫生机构绩效管理的方法，向临床医生和寻求服务的患者们提供知识。

此外，为确保各地均可获得清晰明确的知识，公共卫生主任可以与下列各方面进行合作：

- 公共图书馆；
- 各种社会服务机构；
- 志愿组织和社区组织等第三方机构。

■ 思考题

- 如果赋予您首席知识官的职责和必要权限，那么您的头三项行动是什么？
- 互联网作为人群知识管理的手段，如何能被更好地利用？

—— 参考文献 ——

(7) Moore MH. Creating Public Value: Strategic Management in Government. Boston: Harvard University Press; 1995.

(8) Gray JAM. Where is the Chief Knowledge Officer? BMJ. 1998; 317: 832–833.

(9) Lyons RF. Using evidence: Advances and debates in bridging health research and action. Atlantic Health Promotion Research Centre. 2010: 12.

(10) Gray JAM. Evidence-Based Healthcare and Public Health. London: Elsevier; 2008.

(11) British Standards Institution. Guide to Good Practice in Knowledge Management. London: BSI; 2001.

(12) Resolution adopted by the General Assembly: The human right to water and sanitation. United Nations General Assembly Website http://www.un.org/waterforlifedecade/human_right_to_water.shtml Updated July 2014. Accessed July 23, 2014.

3.4 Creating budgets for populations

In this section, we explore:
- *how population medicine programme budgeting provides a context to encourage decision-making to maximise value*
- *the resources that need to be included in a programme or system budget*
- *how to build a budget even if the finance is in different parts of the health service*
- *how to create a budget and estimate spend even if financial data are not available*
- *steps that can be taken to increase value*

Budget: The contents of a bag or wallet ... A statement of the probable revenue and expenditure for the forthcoming year.
Shorter Oxford English Dictionary

The meaning of the term 'a budget' includes other resources in addition to financial resources. A budget is not a synonym for healthcare finance. Thus, the resources available to a clinician practising population medicine are greater than the financial resources of the service for which they may be managerially responsible because the potential resources include the contributions of volunteers, carers and patients (see Figure 3.5).

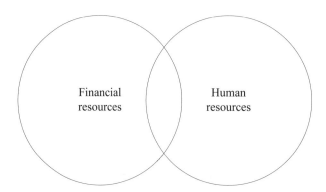

Figure 3.5   The resources for healthcare

It is important for clinicians practising population medicine to be good stewards of all resources irrespective of whether the resources they are responsible for committing are directly charged to their budget (see Figure 3.6). Types of expenditure that tend not to be directly charged to clinical budgets include laboratory tests or imaging.

第 4 节　为人群制订预算

在本节中，我们将探讨：

- 群医学项目预算编制如何为鼓励决策价值最大化营造氛围；
- 项目预算或系统预算需包括的资源；
- 如果财政资源分布在不同的医疗领域里，该如何编制预算；
- 如果无法获得财务数据，该如何编制预算并估算支出；
- 增加价值应采取的步骤。

> 预算：袋子里或钱包里的东西……下一年可能的收入和支出报表。
>
> ——《简明牛津英语字典》

"预算"一词的含义也包括除财务资源外的其他资源。预算并不是医疗融资的代名词。因此，从事群医学的临床医生可利用的资源往往多于机构的财务资源，还有可能来自于志愿者、医疗卫生保健人员和患者的贡献（图 3.5）。

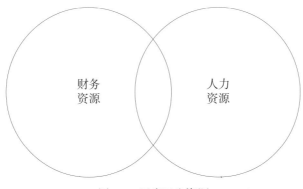

图 3.5　医疗卫生资源

对于从事群医学的临床医生来说，重要的是做好所有资源的统筹管理，无论他们所负责的资源是否直接纳入预算（图 3.6）。通常未直接纳入临床预算的支出类型包括实验室检验或影像学检查。

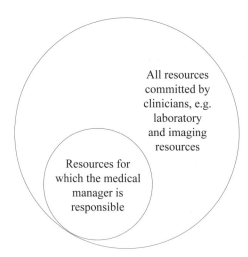

Figure 3.6   Direct and indirect responsibility for resources in a health service

■ Leadership and budget management

The creation of population medicine is a leadership and not a managerial task. It is primarily concerned with culture change and not bureaucratic control.

The key considerations for clinicians responsible for systems of care are:

1.the population they serve, not just the patients referred

2.the need to be good stewards of all the resources already available before they bid for increased resources

3.the need to be part of a community of practice, all of whose members and their resources need to be treated with respect and altruism

Medical managers usually have responsibility for, and authority over, a delegated budget. As shown in Figures 3.5 and 3.6, clinicians with responsibility for a population need to mobilise both financial and human resources over which they have no direct managerial control.

■ Programme budgets

A programme consists of a set of systems with a common knowledge base and a common budget. Programme budgeting is a technique that enables personnel in a health service to identify how much money has been invested in major health programmes, with a view to making future investment decisions more rational and have a greater focus on value.

While the terms 'budgeting' and 'budgets' are normally applied to current and/or future allocations of expenditure, in the context of programme budgeting and programme budgets, it is assumed that they

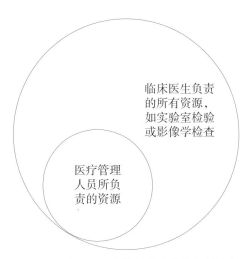

图 3.6 医疗卫生服务资源的直接与间接责任

■ 领导力和预算管理

群医学中的创新行动是领导力的体现，而非一项管理任务。它主要关注的是文化转变，而非行政管控。负责医疗卫生保健系统的临床医生应考虑的关键因素有：

1. 接受医疗的人群，而不只是转诊来的患者；

2. 在争取到新增资源之前需要管理好所有可用资源；

3. 需要成为社区实践工作中的一员，尊重社区中所有成员和资源并遵守"利他"原则。

医疗管理者通常有责任也有权力管理划拨预算。如图 3.5 和图 3.6 所示，负责某个人群的临床医生还需要调动不由自己直接管控的财务和人力资源。

■ 项目预算

项目由包括常识知识库和一般预算在内一套体系组成。编制项目预算是一门技术活，可使医疗卫生人员明确在重大医疗卫生项目中投入了多少资金，以期今后的投资决策更加合理并更注重价值。

虽然"预算编制"和"预算"一词通常适用于目前和／或未来的支出分配，但在项目预算编制和项目预算的语境中，它们也可用

can be applied to past allocations as well. The principle underlying programme budgeting is very simple. If decisions are to be made about broadly defined health-care objectives and priorities – for example, what are the objectives associated with care of the elderly? What relative priorities are attached to the treatment of cancer compared with the prevention of heart disease? – then data should be provided in similarly broad terms to match the nature of the choices. (1)

The NHS in England is fortunate because it has one of the best national programme budget schemes in the world, first initiated in 2002. At the time of writing, there are 23 programme budgets in NHS England, based on the World Health Organization's International Classification of Diseases 10 (ICD10).

This information provides the NHS with an opportunity unique among countries with developed economies to identify:

- *where resources are currently being invested*
- *the value of those investments by relating outcomes to resources*
- *the most effective way of investing in health services in future in relation to the needs of the population*

Estimated expenditure for 2010/11 on each programme in NHS England is set out in Table 1.2 (see section 1.4).

The advantages of programme budgeting are:

- *the potential to engage clinicians in discussions about value for money when conventional budgetary procedures have failed*
- *increased involvement of clinicians in resource allocation*
- *improved information support during decision-making by those who pay for or commission healthcare*
- *the potential to involve the public and patients in decisions about resource allocation*

One weakness associated with programme budgeting is the underlying assumption that people have a single diagnosis. As many people have more than one diagnosis, it is useful to base programme budgets on populations, such as frail elderly people, as well as on conditions (see Figure 3.7).

Overall, data from programme budgeting schemes are very useful. Programme budgeting information enables the clinician responsible for population medicine to improve healthcare for the local population. To ensure the usefulness of the data, however, they need to be:

- *reproduced at the level at which resources are actually allocated, as well as at the national level*
- *related to outcome*

于过去的款项配置。项目预算编制的潜在基本原则非常简单。如果依据宽泛的医疗卫生保健目标和优先项目做出决定，那么提供的数据的广泛程度应该与各项选择相匹配。例如"照护老年人的目标是什么？与预防心脏病相比，癌症治疗方面有哪些相对优先事项？"[1]。

英国国家医疗服务体系（NHS）幸运地拥有世界上最好的国家项目预算方案之一。该方案制定于 2002 年。在撰写本书时，根据世界卫生组织的国际疾病分类第十次修订本（ICD-10），NHS 已有 23 个项目预算。这些信息为 NHS 提供了一个在发达国家中独一无二的机会来明确以下问题：

- 目前正在哪里投入资源；
- 将资源与结局挂钩后的投资价值；
- 与人群需求相关的未来医疗卫生保健服务的最有效投资方式。

表 1.2 列出了 2010/2011 年度 NHS 各项目的预算开支（见第 1 章第 4 节）。项目预算的优点有：

- 当常规预算程序未得到有效执行时，可让临床医生参与投资价值的讨论；
- 提升临床医生对资源分配工作的参与度；
- 加强医疗卫生保健支付者或受委托人在决策过程中的信息支持；
- 为公众和患者参与资源分配决策创造条件。

项目预算的一个缺点是：它假设人们只有单一疾病的诊断。然而，由于很多人被诊断患有一种以上的疾病，基于人群或某些疾病编制预算将有所助益，例如可针对年老体弱者（图 3.7）。

总之，来自项目预算方案的数据非常有用。项目预算信息可使群医学医生改善当地人群的医疗卫生保健状况。然而，为了充分利用数据，这些数据还需要：

- 在资源实际分配层面及国家层面完全一致；
- 与结局相关；

• owned by the clinicians who commit the resources

• further subdivided by systems

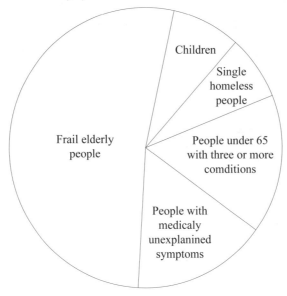

Figure 3.7   Population-based programmes of care

■ System-specific budgets

Whereas a programme is at the level of Cancers and Tumours, Mental Health Disorders or Problems of the Respiratory System, the system is at a finer level of granularity. To take respiratory health as an example, within that programme there are systems of care for asthma, COPD, and sleep apnoea.

Therefore, the person responsible for a population-based programme almost always has an additional responsibility for several population-based systems of care. Furthermore, each of the systems within a programme may be championed by a clinician keen to develop the system for which they are responsible. Thus, the person responsible for a population-based programme not only has to compete with other programmes either to increase resources or to prevent resources being taken away, they also have to deal with competing claims from clinicians responsible for the systems of care within that programme (see Figure 3.8).

People who commission or pay for healthcare must make decisions about the allocation of resources to different programmes, addressing questions such as:

• Should we switch resources from one programme to another?

• Into which programme should we invest new resources?

• From which programme should we cut resources?

- 由负责统筹资源的临床医生所拥有；
- 按系统进一步细分；

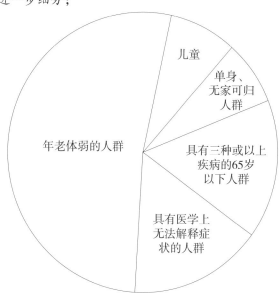

图 3.7 以人群为基础的医疗项目

■ 体系的特定预算

项目是建立在癌症和肿瘤、精神卫生疾病或呼吸系统问题这样的层面上，而体系则是建立在更细化的层面。例如，呼吸系统健康项目包括了哮喘、慢性阻塞性肺疾病和睡眠呼吸暂停综合征在内的多个医疗卫生保健系统。

因此，以人群为基础的项目负责人总是需要对一些以人群为基础的医疗卫生保健系统负有额外责任。此外，临床医生热衷于建设自己负责的体系，项目中的任一系统都可能得到他们的倡导。因此，以人群为基础的项目负责人不仅需要与其他项目竞争，以拉来资源或防止资源流失，还必须要处理好项目内部负责各医疗系统的医生相互竞争的主张（图 3.8）。

医疗卫生保健的支付者或委托人必须决定不同项目之间的资源分配并解决以下问题：

- 我们应该把资源从一个项目转到另一个项目吗？
- 我们应该为哪个项目投入新资源？
- 我们应该从哪个项目削减资源？

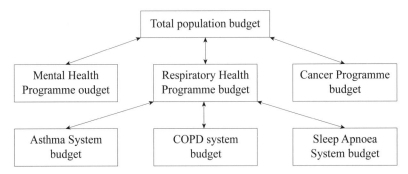

Figure 3.8   Programme and system budgets

Once the budget has been allocated to a programme, however, the clinician practising population medicine has to ask an analogous set of questions.

- *Have we got the distribution of resources right among the various systems of care within the programme or should we redistribute?*
- *If I have to make a cut from one of the services, which should it be?*
- *If I am able to release some resources, to which of the services should those resources be given?*

When practising population medicine, it is essential to be aware of all the key resources that are being spent on a particular condition or a group of conditions within the population served, irrespective of which institutions are responsible for the management of those resources. Rarely is a financial budget for a system available at a local level. Usually it has to be created using the framework in Table 3.4. The simplest approach is to prepare an inventory of all the key resources used, and once they have been listed to express the financial costs of those resources; if there are no accurate costings available, then it is important to make an estimate.

Sometimes, it is relatively easy to identify the financial spend and the use of resources on a specific condition if the service is discrete. In some specialties, however, clinicians will deal with more that one condition during the same clinic, and in primary care the general practitioner will deal with many conditions during the course of one surgery, from asthma to depression to heart failure to a medically unexplained symptom. Despite this, it should be possible to estimate to the nearest million dollars what money is spent on a particular condition in a particular population. Estimates for services delivered to subgroups of that population, such as children or frail elderly people, are more difficult to compile but should still be attempted.

The expenditure associated with calculating to the nearest dollar the amount of money entailed in the delivery of a service is high. Any service in which an attempt is made to bill every item needs to spend a large amount on administration unless it is a specialist hospital doing only elective surgery on healthy people. The precise costing of a single episode of care, or the precise costing of a whole

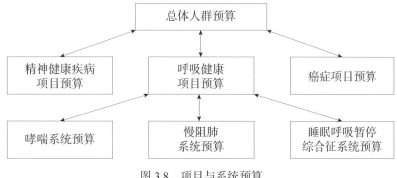

图 3.8 项目与系统预算

若某个项目获得了预算，那么群医学医生必须考虑以下类似的问题：

• 资源是否已在项目内各医疗保健体系之间正确分配，还是应该重新分配？

• 如果必须从中削减一项服务，应该削减哪一项？

• 如果我能够支配一些资源，那么这些资源应该分给哪些服务项目？

在群医学实践中，无论由哪个机构负责管理资源，都必须了解分配给特定疾病或特定患者人群的所有重要资源。一个仅于当地的体系很少能得到财政预算。编制系统预算通常要依据表 3.4 中的框架。最简单的方法就是准备一份清单，列明所使用的全部重要资源，财务成本也就随之明朗；若得不到准确的成本核算，就应该进行估算。

有时，如果各类医疗照护互不相干，确定特定疾病的财务支出和资源利用还是相对容易的。然而，某些专科的临床医生会在同一诊所处理多种医疗问题；初级保健的全科医生会在一次应诊过程中处理多种疾病，如从哮喘到抑郁到心力衰竭再到医学上无法解释的症状。尽管如此，对特定人群特定疾病编制的经费估算应该可以精确到百万美元；而对人群中某些群体（如儿童或年老体弱者）来说，编制医疗预算难度更大但仍需尝试进行。

计算医疗花费的精确数字本身就需要很高的成本。任何医疗机构在试图列出每一条账单细目时都需要耗费大量的管理资源，除非这所医院是一家特殊的专科医院，只为健康人做选择性手术[①]。收集单项或整个医疗卫生保健的

[①] 健康的人不存在复杂的健康状态，这种"理想化"的医院只需要考虑特定手术的成本，医疗花费很容易核算。

service, would not justify the level of expenditure on data collection except as a research exercise. Any service that has to deal with emergencies, or admits older people with four or more diagnoses, would face huge costs were it to try to account for every catheter or drip set. One of the joint winners of the Nobel Prize for Economics in 2009, Oliver Williamson, was recognised for his work over the last 20 years, which highlighted the large transaction costs associated with both markets and bureaucracies when they try to achieve greater efficiency through micro-management.

■ Budget-building: key questions about key resources

The remainder of this section is dedicated to outlining the steps that can be taken to build a budget by mapping all the key resources, both human and financial, that are necessary for a system of care (see Table 3.4).

Building a budget, even if precise financial data are not available, is essential; it is better to be accurate than precise. Accuracy allows clinicians to focus their attention and use their clinical knowledge to obtain increased value from the resources available by asking the following questions, and answering them honestly.

- *Could we reallocate the resources among the services funded by the programme to achieve increased value for the common problems we face?*
- *Within the budget for each common problem, can we shift resources from lower- to higher-value interventions?*
- *Of the activities we do, can we reduce the level of one or more to free resources?*
- *Could we reduce the purchase cost of some drugs or equipment?*

Thus, value can be increased by addressing these questions and acting upon the answers.

■ Questions for reflection

- *How would you organise your first meeting on population-based planning?*
- *How should common symptoms such as breathlessness be dealt with in a programme budgeting system that assumes every patient has a diagnosis?*
- *If you were a commissioner faced by a demand for more resources for cataract surgery, how could you relate this bid to other uses within an eye service to which the same amount of resources could be put?*

References

(1) Mooney GH, Russell EM, Weir RD. Choices for Health Care.

精确成本数据不能用来判断支出水平，除非是用于实验研究。若将收费精确到每一支导管或每一个输液装置，任何急诊或接诊患有四种及以上疾病老年人的医疗活动都将产生巨大开销。2009 年诺贝尔经济学奖的共同获奖者之一奥利弗·威廉姆森因其过去 20 年的工作而得到认可。他的研究强调，市场和行政机构试图通过微观管理以获得更大效益时将会产生巨额交易成本。

■ 预算编制：与重要资源有关的关键问题

本节剩余部分将通过提供医疗卫生保健系统所需人力和财政的全部重要资源的信息，专门对预算编制的步骤做出概述（表 3.4）。

即使得不到精确的财务数据，也有必要进行预算编制；预算的准确性比精确性更重要。准确的预算可以使临床医生集中精力，通过提出并诚实回答以下问题，应用自己的临床知识从可用资源中获取更多价值：

- 我们能否重新分配项目资助的资源，为面临的常见问题实现增值？
- 在每个常见问题的预算范围内，我们能否将资源从价值较低的干预措施转移到价值较高的？
- 在我们所进行的各项活动中，是否可以降低一项或多项活动的水准以节约资源？
- 我们能否降低某些药品或设备的采购成本？

因此，通过解决上述问题并将答案付诸行动，就能实现增值。

■ 思考题

- 你将如何组织第一次以人群为基础的规划会议？
- 在假定每个患者都有一种疾病的项目预算系统中，应该如何处理像呼吸困难这样常见症状？
- 若你是一名委员，当白内障手术有更多的资源需求时，你如何将这一需求与同等资源但用于其他眼科服务的内容结合起来一并进行考虑呢？

────────────────────────── 参考文献 ─

London: The Macmillan Press Ltd; 1980: 10–11.

Table 3.4 Budget-building: key questions about key resources

Key resource	Comment	Key questions	Key financial issues
Patients	Patients are probably the most neglected resource.	• What steps are being taken to provide and support self-care? • Do the patients hold their own records? • Can patients request follow-up consultations or telephone advice as they feel they require it, or are they scheduled into regular clinic appointments?	Probably no finance identified for patients; there should be a budget for patient information; if there is none, one should be created.
Carers	Carers are another neglected resource.	• How heavy is the burden on carers? • Does carer exhaustion play any part in demand on services? • Do carers have all the information they need, including information about access in an emergency?	No finance usually identified for carers; as for patients, there should be a budget for carer information.
Patient organisations	Patient organisations play an invaluable role in networks of care.	• How many national patient organisations are there? • How many, if any, local branches are there of these organisations? • What is the potential for strengthening and expanding their contribution?	Patient and carer organisations can be helped without finance, e.g. by the offer of rooms for meetings, but small grants give a very good return on investment in patient organisations.
General practice	There is a high degree of variation in the clinical practice of general practitioners.	• What proportion of general practitioners' time is spent on this condition? • What resources do general practitioners feel they lack? • Are there particular general practitioners with special skills or interests who want to do more? • Could general practice trainees be more involved with the service?	The only way to estimate the financial cost of general practice time is to take the percentage of consultations on the condition and use this to calculate the financial cost of general practice input; this estimate is probably not worth the effort required.

表 3.4　预算编制：与重要资源有关的关键问题

重要资源	解释	关键问题	关键的财务问题
患者	患者是最可能被忽视的资源	• 正在采取哪些措施支持自我保健？ • 患者是否持有自己的健康档案？ • 如果患者需要，是否可以请求随诊或电话咨询，或安排到常规的预约门诊？	可能没有固定为患者所用的经费；应该编制患者信息的预算；如果没有，则应该编制此类预算
医疗照护人员	医疗照护人员是另外一类被忽视的资源	• 医疗照护人员的负担有多重？ • 医疗照护人员的过度疲劳会对医疗需求有影响吗？ • 医疗照护人员有他们所需要的全部信息吗，包括急诊的就诊信息？	通常没有针对医疗照护人员的经费；如同患者一样，应该编制与卫生保健人员信息相关的预算
患者组织	患者组织在保健网络中发挥着不可估量的作用	• 国家级的患者组织有多少？ • 如果有国家级的患者组织，这些组织在地方上有多少分支机构？ • 加强和扩张其作用的潜在好处是什么？	患者和医疗照护人员组织可以得到除经费之外的帮助，如提供会议室。如对患者组织提供小额经费，必定能得到很好的投资回报
全科医生	全科医生的临床实践有着很大程度的差异	• 在这种情况下，全科医生花费时间占多大比例？ • 全科医生认为他们缺少什么资源？ • 那些具有专长或对某些方向感兴趣的全科医生想做更多工作吗？ • 接受全科培训的人员可以更多地参与这项服务吗？	现有条件下，用就诊时间所占比例这一指标是估算全科医师时间成本的唯一方法，以此还可用于计算全科诊疗投入的财务成本；然而为此类估算投入如此多的精力可能不足为法

continued

Key resource	Comment	Key questions	Key financial issues

Community services	Community services may be based in a community services organisation or work as outreach services from a hospital.	• What is the involvement of:
		  –health visitors;
		  –home nurses;
		  –occupational therapists;
		  –physiotherapists;
		  –podiatrists.
		• What constrains do these staff face in delivering high value care?
		• Who are the leaders within these professional groups?
			Good data on number of visits and work done, but financial cost may have to be estimated by using the percentage of work done on the condition in relation to the total budget of community services.

Social care	Social care is a key resource even though it may be supported from another financial stream.	• How much resource does social care invest in people with this condition? • What constraints impair social services' ability to be as helpful as the health service thinks they could be? • In what way could healthcare resources be used to reduce pressure on social care budgets?	Usually very well costed by the local authority.
Private care	Private care has more relevance for some health services than others; impacts on health service resources can be both positive and negative.	• What private sector resources are used by people with this condition? • Is the impact on publicly funded services negative or positive? • How could a clearer understanding between sectors improve the value derived from public resources?	The cost per case, or at least the price charged, is usually public knowledge; the number of cases is not.
Pharmacists	The knowledge and skills of pharmacists are probably the most under-used in the healthcare workforce.	• How much hospital or specialist pharmacist time is committed to the programme? • Is there a pharmacist with a special interest or responsibility? • Could the specialist pharmacist make an even more valuable contribution? • How many community pharmacists are involved with patients? • Could their contribution be more valuable with additional training or specialisation?	It is usually simple to cost whole-time equivalents using pharmacists' salaries.

续表

重要资源	解释	关键问题	关键的财务问题
社区服务	社区服务可以来自社区医疗机构或来自医院的外展服务	• 涉及的方面： 　– 保健访视员 　– 家庭护士 　– 职业治疗师 　– 理疗师 　– 足病治疗师 • 这些工作人员在提供高价值照护服务时会遇到哪些限制？ • 这些专业团体中的领导者是谁？	尽管已经有了关于访视次数和已完成工作的高质量数据，但是财务成本可能还需要通过与社区服务总预算相关工作和完成的百分比来估算
社会关怀	即使社会关怀的资金支持可能来源于其他渠道，它仍然是一项重要的资源	• 社会关怀为患病人群投入了多少资源？ • 哪些制约因削弱了本应和医疗机构发挥相同作用的社会服务机构的能力？ • 医疗保健资源可以采用哪种方式来减轻社会关怀的预算压力？	通常是由地方政府全部承担
私人医疗保健	私人医疗保健与某些医疗服务的关系更紧密：对医疗服务资源的影响可能是积极的，也可能是消极的	• 此种情况的人群都可以使用哪些私人部门的资源？ • 公共资助医疗服务产生的是消极影响还是积极影响？ • 如何通过各部门之间的充分理解来提高公共资源的价值？	通常每个病例的花费或起步价收费是众所周知的，但病例数量并不清楚
药剂师	药剂师的知识和技能可能是医疗保健人员中发挥作用最不充分的	• 医院药剂师或专业药剂师为项目投入了多少时间？ • 是否有特殊兴趣或责任的药剂师？ • 专科药剂师能做出更有价值的贡献吗？ • 有多少社区的药剂师是为患者服务的？ • 额外培训或专业课程是否会使他们的付出更有价值？	用药剂师的工资来衡量其全职工作成本通常是比较容易的

continued

Key resource	Comment	Key questions	Key financial issues
Medication	Medication is often the fastest growing cost.	• How many people receive drug treatment? • How much variation is there in prescribing? • Are generic options available and what proportion of prescriptions are generic? • What proportion of drugs is taken as prescribed?	Usually well documented.
Specialist clinics	The term "outpatients" is an outdated 19th century term.	• How many clinic sessions are there in the year? −Are all the sessions managed by consultants? −Assuming a 100% attendance rate, how many consultations can take place in these sessions? −Are telephone or email consultations and contacts available?	Much more difficult to find data; clinics may not be charged to each specialist service.
Hospital beds	Even though hospital beds are not owned by the relevant specialty, an estimate of bed days should be included in the inventory.	• What is the average duration of stay? • How many admissions take place in the course of the year? • How many bed days are used in the year? • What proportion of hospital admissions were day cases?	Difficult to cost but the finance department are usually able to provide an estimate.
Theatre resources	Theatre resources are not applicable to every specialty; they are often difficult to calculate because the relevant operations may be done as part of a long list with other operations.	• How many operations were done in the last year? • What was the cost of equipment used in the operations?	The theatre manager can often provide good costings for a theatre session.
Imaging	For some diseases, the demand for imaging is growing at a faster rate than that for drugs	• Number of MRIs and rate of increase since previous year. • Number of CTs and rate of increase since previous year. • Number of other images and increase since previous year. • Is there any scope for increasing interventional techniques to reduce the use of other resources?	Some imaging departments have good costings.

续表

重要资源	解释	关键问题	关键的财务问题
治疗药物	治疗药物往往是增长最快的成本	• 有多少人接受药物治疗？ • 处方有多大差别？ • 是否有通用处方，占多大比例？ • 按处方服药的比例是多少？	通常有完整的记录
专科诊所	"门诊患者"是一个过时的19世纪术语	• 一年有多少次会诊？ 　– 所有的会诊都由高年资医师负责吗？ 　– 假设会诊的参与率为100%，在这些会诊中有多少次能够进行专业咨询讨论？ 　– 患者可以用电话或电子邮件方式咨询和联系医生吗？	很难找到相关数据；诊所可能并不向每项专科服务收费
医院床位	尽管病床不归相关专科所有，但财产清单中应包括床位使用天数的估算	• 平均住院时间是多少？ • 一年中办理住院次数有多少？ • 一年内住院日有多少天？ • 住院患者中门诊患者所占比例是多少？	虽然很难计算成本，但财务部门通常还是能够提供预算
手术室资源	手术室资源并不适用于每个专科；有些手术可能需要与其他手术联合完成。通常很难计算	• 去年做了多少台手术？ • 在手术中使用设备的费用是多少？	手术室管理者通常应提供合理的手术室成本核算
影像学检查	某些疾病对影像学检查需求的增长速度快于对药物的需求	• 磁共振成像检查的数量以及与往年相比的增长率 • CT检查的数量以及与往年相比的增长率。 • 其他影像学检查的数量以及与往年相比的增长率 • 是否存在以增加技术干预措施来减少其他资源的使用？	有些影像部门有合理的成本核算

continued

Key resource	Comment	Key questions	Key financial issues
Laboratory services	More than one estimate may need to be prepared for different types of service, e.g. biochemistry and haematology, depending on the condition.	• Where are the tests most commonly ordered? • Is it possible to classify the tests as used for either diagnostic or monitoring purposes? • What are the rates of increase in the five most commonly requested tests?	The cost per test may be available but remember to cost the work generated by false-positive test results.

Specialist personnel	Specialist personnel are the most valuable and expensive resource.	• How many whole-time equivalents of:
		  –nursing staff?
		  –medical staff?
		  –physiotherapists?
		  –occupational therapists
		  –scientists?
		  –managerial staff?
		  –staff in training?
			The cost can be estimated from the salaries of specialist staff.

Real estate	Real estate comprises such items as wards, clinics, and offices; at present, real estate is rarely charged to clinical teams, but this will change.	• How much space is occupied by the service as sole occupier? • How much space do we share with other services? • Of the space we occupy alone, what proportion of it is not occupied for more than half the time?	Difficult to estimate but can be done by using the proportion of the whole hospital budget that the service represents and then calculating the proportion of the capital value.
Information Technology (IT)	Although IT is a consumer of resources, it is also a potential saver of resources.	• Does the service have any contracts for IT? • What proportion of the total IT budget is the service responsible for?	The possibility of costing IT depends on the balance of stand-alone IT to the share of general hospital IT.
Management and administration	It is essential to maximise productivity in management and administration, but what is the right level of investment?	• Number of whole-time equivalent administrative and management staff. • Notional share of central management costs, e.g. human resource departments. • Number of whole-time equivalents of professional staff with explicit management duties.	Staff wholly employed in the service can be calculated; general overheads can be estimated as 50% of clinical staff salaries.

续表

重要资源	解释	关键问题	关键的财务问题
实验室服务	根据不同的疾病，可能需要对不同类型的实验室服务（如生物化学和血液学）进行多次评估	• 实验室检查最常由哪个部门提出？ • 可以将检查分为用于诊断目的或者用于监测目的的两大类吗？ • 五种最常见检测项目的增长率是多少？	每次检测的成本是可以核算的，但也须包括假阳性检测结果的成本
专家	专家是最宝贵和最昂贵的资源	• 各种全职的专家人数有多少： – 护理专家 – 医学专家 – 物理治疗师 – 职业治疗师 – 实验室专家 – 管理人员 – 接受培训的人员	人员的成本可用专家的工资来进行估算
不动产	不动产包括病房、诊所和办公室等；目前，不动产的费用很少由临床团队承担，但这种情况可能会改变	• 有多少空间是完全被使用者单独占用了？ • 与其他服务共享的空间有多少？ • 在独占的空间中，使用时间不超过一半的比例是多少？	尽管难以估算不动产的成本，但可以通过某项服务在整个医院预算中所占的比例来进行估算，然后再计算实际固定资本价值所占的比例
信息技术	虽然信息技术是资源的消耗者，但也可以是资源的潜在节约者	• 服务项目与信息技术方面有合同吗？ • 在总的信息技术预算中，该信息技术服务所占的比例是多少？	是否能对信息技术成本进行核算，取决于独立的信息技术与医院综合信息技术共享的程度
管理与行政	最大限度地提高管理和行政的运行效率至关重要，但是合理的投资力度应该是多少？	• 全职行政和管理人员数 • 中央管理成本中的名义成本份额，例如人力资源部门 • 具有明确管理职责的全职专业人员数	全部受雇于该服务的工作人员的成本是可以核算的；日常管理费可用临床工作者工资的 50% 进行估算

Coda The new paradigm: population and personalised medicine

Population and personalised medicine is a call to be expert at individual and population care. Every clinician and manager must be expert in three jobs: the (clinical) job they do (for the individual), improving that job, and working for the good of the population.

For the last four decades, the paradigm of healthcare has focused on effectiveness, quality, and safety, primarily involving clinicians and institutions. A new paradigm is emerging, however, driven by the economic crisis, the Internet and, to a lesser degree, the human genome project. The primary focus is now on value for populations and individuals.

Even within one country questions about most of the common diseases cannot be answered, such as:

- *Is the service for people with seizures and epilepsy better in Auckland than in Wellington?*
- *How many liver disease services are there in Australia, and how many should there be?*
- *Which service for frail elderly people in the Auckland area provides the best value?*
- *Which service for people with bipolar disorder improved most in the last year?*

We know to the nearest dollar what we spend on every hospital but not to the nearest one hundred million dollars what we spend on epilepsy or breathlessness. We need personalised healthcare, to maximise value for individuals, and population healthcare.

Population healthcare focuses primarily on populations defined by a common need, which may be a symptom such as breathlessness, a condition such as arthritis, or a common characteristic such as frailty in old age. It does not focus on institutions, specialties, or technologies. Its aim is to maximise value for those populations and the individuals within them, and clinicians practising population medicine can and must play a leading part in its creation.

结语 新的范式：群医学及个体医学

群医学及个体医学呼吁在医疗保健领域里"成为个体及群体两方面的专家"。每一名临床医生和管理者都必须精通三项工作：所从事的（临床）工作（针对个体）、改进本职工作和为增进人群福祉而努力。

在过去四十年里，医疗卫生范式一直关注医疗的有效性、质量和安全性，主要涉及临床医生及医疗卫生机构。然而，在经济危机、互联网以及人类基因组计划或多或少的推动下，一种新的范式正在兴起。这种范式目前主要关注的是群体和个体的价值。

即使在一个国家内，大多数常见疾病的问题也无法解答，例如：

- 奥克兰是否为癫痫患者提供了优于惠灵顿的医疗服务？

- 在澳大利亚有多少为肝脏患者提供的医疗服务，应该有多少？

- 哪项服务对奥克兰地区的年老体弱者最有价值？

- 在过去一年中，哪一项为双相情感障碍患者提供的医疗服务改善最多？

我们能将为每家医院投入的资金精确到 1 美元，在癫痫和呼吸困难上的花费却无法精确到百万美元。我们需要个性化的医疗卫生保健，使个体及群体医疗保健的价值最大化。

群医学主要关注有共同需求的人群，这些需求可能是像呼吸困难这样的症状，也可能是像关节炎这样的疾病，还可能是像老年体弱这种共同的特征。它的关注点不在机构、专科或技术。其目的是使这些人群以及其中个体获得最大的医疗卫生服务价值，而群医学医生能够而且必须在这一过程中发挥主导作用。